Nourishing Menopause:

The Whole-Food Guide

to Balancing

Your Hormones

Naturally

By

Margie King, J.D., M.B.A.
Holistic Menopause Health Coach

Publisher's Note

This book is not intended as a substitute for medical advice from a physician. The material contained herein is for general information and for the purpose of educating individuals on nutrition, lifestyle, health and fitness, and related topics. Consult with a physician or other qualified healthcare provider before embarking on any new treatment, diet, fitness or exercise program. Any personal stories shared in this book are personal to the users and will not be typical of the results you will have if you apply the information provided in this book. The author and publisher specifically disclaim any liability for loss or risk, personal or otherwise, incurred as a direct or indirect consequence of the use and application of the contents of this book.

The information and recommendations provided in this book have not been evaluated by the Food and Drug Administration and are provided for educational purposes only.

Contents

Introduction

"I am not a has-been, I'm a will-be."

– Lauren Bacall

My own menopause journey has been going on for 20 years. Today I've settled into my comfortable and thriving post-menopause years. But it hasn't always been so peaceful and my body certainly didn't go willingly through "The Change."

Throughout my 40's I was going through peri-menopause. It started with occasional hot flashes. But then I developed fibroids that gave me a distended belly. My monthly bleeding was so heavy, I had to wear two tampons AND a maxi-pad and change them every 45 minutes. There was no predicting when I would start leaking and staining.

I was afraid to go anywhere because I might not make it to a bathroom on a moment's notice. I was a prisoner in my own house for two days every month.

My doctors wanted me to have a hysterectomy. The fibroids were growing so quickly they were afraid I had a uterine sarcoma, which is an incurable and deadly cancer. It was a shock to me because I had never been really sick in my life and now I was being told I might have an incurable disease. It was a real wake-up call.

I didn't like the options the doctors were giving me: major surgery or the risk of a deadly cancer. At the same time I was dealing with hot flashes, night sweats and low energy.

I started doing my own research beginning with Dr. Christiane Northrup, who wrote *"The Wisdom of Menopause"* and found that there were things that I could do for myself just by adjusting my diet. I read everything that I could get my hands on and started experimenting on myself.

By increasing the fiber in my diet I began to combat the estrogen imbalance in my body. Did you know that fiber can affect your estrogen levels? Most people don't.

I also learned what other foods were especially beneficial in menopause and I started to get the sugar out of my diet. I collected more and more research and put it all together in a plan.

Following my own plan, I started losing weight. After a year when I returned to the doctor, my fibroids had not only stabilized, they were shrinking. Also, my menopause symptoms all improved – I had fewer hot flashes and I was sleeping better with fewer night sweats.

I was determined to go through menopause naturally without drugs or hormones or surgery. I did it and now my mission is to teach other women to use the power of food to support their own hormonal system.

That's why I wrote this book. I want you to be able to take charge of your life and your menopause symptoms. I want you to stop feeling like a victim and stop treating your body as though it were the enemy.

I wish I knew then what I know now. That's why I'm hoping that you can take advantage of my experience.

You don't have to go through menopause in the dark.

In this book, you'll find the information you need to take back your life and navigate "The Change" naturally.

Here is just some of what you'll find in these pages:

- How to set your intentions for a fulfilling menopause
- The power of positive affirmations
- How to manage your metabolic fire to burn more calories
- The keys to dietary fats: good, bad and ugly
- Why we gain weight at midlife
- Controlling insulin to control weight
- Carbohydrates and weight loss
- Why we have mood swings at menopause
- Beating mood swings and depression
- The food/mood connection
- Five bad mood foods to avoid

3

- Primary foods: Nourishment not on a plate
- Why soy is not a health food
- Controlling hot flashes and night sweats
- Balancing hormones naturally
- Adrenal fatigue, salt and iodine
- Stress busters
- Protecting your heart and breasts at midlife
- Eating to prevent heart disease
- The magic of magnesium
- Omega-3 and Omega-6 fats
- Food and breast cancer
- Role of vitamin D and iodine in breast cancer
- Xenoestrogens (environmental toxins)
- Eating for bone health
- Calcium supplements: busting the myth
- Vitamin D and magnesium for bone health
- Superfoods for Menopause
- Red wine: pros and cons

This information is powerful and changed my life. It can change your life also - if you let it.

If you're anxious to get started, here are just a few basic concepts that you can use right away:

Quick Start Guide

Here are 5 basic things that you could start doing right now to ease your journey into the sisterhood of wise women.

1. ***Cut out <u>added sugar</u> and refined carbohydrates.*** These can raise insulin levels, promote weight gain and lead to more fat stores, especially around the belly, that promote higher levels of circulating estrogen.

2. ***Add more fruits and vegetables.*** <u>Phytoestrogens</u> are weak plant estrogens found in over 300 plants including blueberries, cherries, cranberries, carrots, bananas, beets, oranges, onions, peppers, oats, plums, olives and potatoes. Phytoestrogens bind to estrogen receptors and balance estrogen levels by having an estrogenic effect if your estrogen levels are too low, and by blocking stronger estrogens if your levels are too high.

3. ***Increase fiber, especially <u>flax seeds</u>.*** Flax seeds are rich in lignans, which are particularly strong phytoestrogens, and have been shown in studies to help in both the prevention and treatment of breast cancer. Lignans not only have anti-viral, anti-bacterial and antioxidant properties but they also help lower LDL (bad) cholesterol and raise HDL (good) cholesterol.

4. ***Avoid caffeine, spicy foods and alcohol***. These are all heat-producing substances and will contribute to hot flashes. Instead, try cooling foods like melon, bean sprouts, celery, apples, asparagus and grapes.

5. ***Only eat <u>organic</u> animal protein and dairy products***. Most animal protein and dairy has been treated with hormones which may compound an estrogen imbalance. Stick with organic meat and dairy which is hormone free.

Chapter 1

A Holistic Approach to Menopause

A holistic approach to menopause means taking this time in our lives to examine how we are doing in all areas of our health and wellness. All parts of our lives are interconnected and no one goes through menopause in a vacuum. And no two women go through menopause in exactly the same way.

The approach of most medical practitioners is to treat a single symptom of menopause or a series of symptoms. A holistic approach treats the whole person. Even with respect to food, a holistic approach does not dwell on calories, carbs, fats, and proteins. The point is not to create lists of restrictions, or good and bad foods. Instead, a holistic approach to health and wellness works to help create a happy, healthy life in a way that is flexible, fun and rewarding.

Whether your health goal is to achieve your optimal weight, reduce food cravings, increase sleep, or maximize your energy, there is one thing that is essential. It's most important to develop a deeper understanding of the food and lifestyle choices that work best for you. Your ultimate goal should be to implement lasting changes that will improve your energy, balance and health.

Women experiencing menopause have a real challenge. It's not a medical challenge although this perfectly normal transition out of the reproductive years has become shamelessly medicalized for the benefit of pharmaceutical companies and the medical industry.

It's more of a cultural challenge. We are bombarded by images of young women – girls really – and told that we have to have smooth skin and pinched waists or else be relegated to the sidelines. Society does not want to see women beyond their youthful years.

In part, that's because women have been so completely sexualized that a women hormonally past her child-bearing years is unworthy of attention and invisible to the eye.

But that's when the fun begins. Women at midlife can live the life that calls them, rather than the life that society demands. That freedom is the biggest blessing of menopause.

This book is not about what society wants women to do. It's about what we know we can do. It's not about women as a market for the big business of hormone replacement therapy. It's not about herbs or creams or any commercial products. You may want to explore those things on your own but it's not what this book is about.

The Power of Food

This book is about the most basic thing that you can do for yourself at midlife. It is about the power of food to nourish us, heal us and make us thrive during menopause.

Why food? For a couple of reasons. One is that we are what we eat. Everything we put in our mouths becomes our blood, skin, bones, brain and even our thoughts and emotions.

Another reason is that food is a powerful "drug" -- more potent than even the hormones in your body.

Elite athletes understand the idea that food fuels their performance but many of us mere mortals don't make the connection. We need to take a page out of their book and realize that we need to be in the best shape possible when we go through menopause.

I don't like to use pugilistic analogies but I'm a product of the streets of Philadelphia and Rocky comes to mind for me. If you saw the movie (the first one is plenty), you know that Rocky trained – seriously trained – before going into the ring.

You have to be in shape to take on a challenge and in this case your challenge is menopause. If you are not in training, you might well get knocked for a loop. But if you are in overall good shape you will be able to cope much better with all the changes that your body is juggling.

I learned this the hard way about 10 years ago when I decided to take a bike trip in Ireland. I had not been on a bike in more than 40 years but it seemed like a great way to see the Emerald Island. Several months before the trip, the tour guide advised me repeatedly to get out on the road and ride at least three times a week to prepare. Did I listen? No. I went to the gym and rode on the stationary bike. Wrong move. I suffered because I did not have the stamina I needed for long rides outside on the open road. I was not in condition and after the first day, I couldn't walk or sit, let alone get back on that bike.

It's the same for menopause. Starting in your 40s, your body goes through something very demanding that requires you to be in best shape possible to minimize its effects. Your training starts with food.

Why Whole Foods Matter

What makes an apple so good for us? Is it the vitamin C? Vitamin K or B6? Is it the soluble fiber or the insoluble fiber? Is it the potassium or the phytosterols?

Or is it the apple? What a concept.

Western science is obsessed with deconstructing food, researching and analyzing its component parts, isolating the "active ingredients," repackaging them in pills or powders and prescribing them in daily doses. But according to Annemarie Colbin, Ph.D., author of *Food and Healing*, this chemistry-based theory of nutrition is completely upside down.

Dr. Colbin, founder and CEO of the Natural Gourmet Institute for Health and Culinary Arts, has crafted her own nutrition theory based on more than 30 years of nutrition practice and teaching. She prefers to liken nutrition to systems theory, and believes that *a whole food, like the human being consuming it, is complex and much greater than the sum of its parts*.

"Whole foods," according to Dr. Colbin are those "foods that nature provides and all the edible parts." She limits them to foods that have one ingredient, such as whole grains, beans, vegetables, fruits, nuts and seeds.

Animal foods are a little trickier to identify. Eggs are a whole food, but steaks are not unless you're eating the entire cow. She includes small fish if you eat the head and bones, and small birds like quail. Whole milk is included but **low-fat** dairy is not.

Why does eating the whole food matter?

Dr. Colbin's theory is that our bodies know the difference between a whole food and an aggregation of isolated nutrients. The human body has evolved over thousands of years to eat the food that nature presents to it. If that food has been split apart or "fragmented," the body knows and goes looking for the missing parts.

For example, Dr. Colbin suggests that if you eat fragmented wheat like white bread, where the bran and germ of the whole grain have been removed, your body will still be hungry and seek the missing part of the food, i.e., something with fiber or crunch. Likewise, health nuts who devour wheat germ or wheat bran in isolation will also feel something is missing and may find themselves craving refined flour in the form of cake at night.

Whole foods help control cravings.

When we eat only part of a food that has been "fragmented," i.e., broken down into its component parts, our bodies know and want what's missing. This can set us up for cravings according to Dr. Colbin.

She cites table sugar as an example. It's a fragmented food taken from the whole food sugar cane. Very little of the sugar cane makes it into the final product. In fact, it's estimated that 17 feet of sugar cane are required to make one cup of sugar.

What's missing is mostly the water content found in natural sugar cane. The result? Sugar makes you thirsty. If you drink sodas, which have about 12 teaspoons of sugar in a serving, you'll be thirsty afterward and continue to drink more soda, creating a vicious cycle.

Fruit juices are another fragmented food. When you drink orange juice, for example, all of the fiber from the fruit is missing and your body will crave something to chew on. This may set you up for a craving for chips or something crunchy. The same is true even if you think you are being really healthy and juicing vegetables.

Why health nuts might crave junk food

In fact, this problem can affect people who are trying to be healthy just as much as people who are eating junk food. For instance, Dr. Colbin warns to be very careful of vitamin and mineral supplements. Although they may have a place at certain times to treat a condition or deficiency, they are also fragments of food. The body may have difficulty processing these isolated nutrients outside of the whole food.

Dr. Colbin suggests that supplements may even make you less likely to want to eat vegetables and set you up for junk food cravings to balance out too many vitamins or minerals. Her advice is to use vitamins and supplements if medically required, but not every day and not forever.

It's all about maintaining the natural balance in the foods that nature provides. And there's no need to worry about striving for perfection or changing your diet radically. Dr. Colbin recommends that you aim for 70% whole foods in your diet to keep everything in balance. Start small, make a few changes, listen to your body and see if you notice a difference.

Bio-Individuality™: There is no one like you!

There is no one right prescription for menopause. Remember as you go through this book that no one way of eating works for everyone. This is a concept called bio-individuality developed by Joshua Rosenthal of the Institute for Integrative Nutrition™. One person's food is another person's poison and that's why fad diets don't work. Each of us is a conglomerate of multiple factors that combine to form a unique organism with unique nutritional needs.

Ancestry is a huge factor. If you have Japanese ancestors you may thrive on a diet of rice, sea vegetables and fish, but you may not be able to tolerate dairy. If, however, you come from a Scandinavian background where dairy is a dietary staple, you may have no problem digesting milk products and in fact may need dairy to thrive.

Your blood type may also have an effect on what foods are compatible with your digestive system. Your type of metabolism is another factor. Later we'll be talking about those things.

Your sex is a factor. Women and men may need different nutrients in different amounts. Age makes a difference. You ate differently when you were a child and a teen, a pregnant or nursing mother. You may also eat differently when you go through menopause.

There are no absolute food rules. Keep in mind that you cannot say that "red meat is bad" or "whole wheat is good." It depends on what individual you are talking about. Always keep the concept of bio-individuality in mind when you hear diet and nutrition advice.

What works for me may not work for you. Throughout this book, I will be making suggestions based on what I have found from my experience and the experience of my clients, but those suggestions may not work for you. I cannot tell you that something is definitely going to make a difference for you.

The only way to know what works for you is to try different things and pay attention to how you feel in your body and what reaction you notice.

Remember to give things a fair chance. Trying something once or twice is not usually sufficient to tell if you will do well on it. When trying something new, give it at least two weeks before passing judgment. You may have to try a food 10 or 12 times to develop a taste for it.

As you go through this book, I hope you will be trying new things and finding an eating plan that is going to be your own individual solution to thriving at midlife.

Recipe: Dijon Vinaigrette

- 1 tablespoon Dijon mustard
- 1/2 cup red wine vinegar
- 1 cup extra virgin olive oil
- Celtic sea salt
- ground black pepper

Whisk ingredients together to emulsify, or shake in a glass jar to combine.

Recipe: Morning Sausage and Kale

- 1 teaspoon extra virgin olive oil or coconut oil
- 1/2 small red onion
- 1 pre-cooked sausage (from pastured animals)
- 1/2 bunch organic kale
- 1 tablespoon balsamic vinaigrette

Slice onion in long thin slivers. Heat oil and sauté onion for 5 minutes. Slice sausage in 1/2 inch rounds and chop kale. Add sausage and kale to pan and cook for 5 minutes. Remove from heat and sprinkle with balsamic vinegar.

Chapter 2

Setting Your Midlife Intention

So often we set out on a new project with a vague notion that it sounds like a good idea. But we don't have any specific goals for all the time that we're investing in a project. It's the same with menopause. You know it's coming and it's going to mean a big change.

What kind of change do you want it to be?

When I set out to write this book, I spent some time setting my intentions for this creation before I put it out into the world. Here's what I came up with:

> *The intention of this book is to change your attitude toward menopause, dispel the myths, and provide empowering health information so you experience this time of your life as vibrant and energetic – your best life ever.*

That's a tall order. For that to happen you have to be willing to change not only physically but also mentally.

My intention is for you to jettison your negative stereotypical thoughts about menopause. You have to lose the negative self-talk that holds you back and makes you unhappy. In order for this to happen *you have to act as though your life depends on it - because it does.*

The truth is that menopause is a wonderful time of transformation. It's a natural phase of development that brings women to a stage of life that can be the most rewarding they have ever known.

The symptoms of menopause are no less than messages from your soul. They signal the unhealthy habits and relationships that you've been putting up with for years. These symptoms force us to look inward and see, sometimes for the first time or with new eyes, our relationships to others, to food, to work, to society and to our own spirit. Do these relationships serve our best interests or do we need to make changes?

What are your own personal goals are for this transformative time of your life? What motivated you to pick up this book? What and how do you want to change? Get clear on that and write down what your objectives are.

Now, are you ready to commit to those objectives?

I'm talking about making a commitment – not to me, or to anyone else – but to yourself and to your future. **You** will be doing the hard work. So make a promise to yourself today.

Banish Negative Thoughts about Menopause

Talking about change is pretty easy, but making it happen is not always so simple. In order for us to have positive feelings about menopause we really have to root out the stereotype of the midlife woman that runs throughout our culture.

What image comes to mind for you when you say or you hear the word "menopause?"

Here are some typical answers:

- Bitch
- Crazy
- Crazy bitch
- Blob
- Moody
- Hot flash
- Angry
- Wrinkled
- Depressed
- Irrational
- Tired
- Sweaty
- Fat
- Dragging
- Invisible
- Dried up
- Exhausted

But there are many advantages to going through menopause. Let's focus on the positive:

- No need for birth control
- Freedom from periods, pads and tampons
- No more monthly cramping
- No more leaking worries
- No more tampon clutter in your purse

Negative stereotypes surrounding menopause abound in our culture. But in other cultures, the idea of a woman with graying hair or past her child-bearing years will evoke other adjectives:

➢ Wise
➢ Nurturing
➢ Spiritual
➢ Calm
➢ Truthful
➢ Steady
➢ Outspoken
➢ Goddess

You can choose how you will think of yourself and your fellow women as you go through these years. It's not always easy because you're fighting the cultural stereotype.

How do you overcome those negative images? You start with your own thoughts.

Daily Affirmations

It takes discipline and practice to change your mind. And it is all about changing your thoughts. We often make the mistake of believing that our thoughts reflect the world we experience, and that thoughts are processing the information we receive from the outside world. But you may be surprised to know that that is not the case.

Our thoughts create our world. Our thoughts are our reality.

That's a big mind shift when you really accept it. You want to pack your mind with positive thoughts and get rid of the negative self-talk. You know what I'm talking about – thoughts like: *I'm not good enough; I don't have enough money; I'm not thin enough; I'm not smart enough; I'm not strong enough.*

What are you telling yourself all day long? If those are your thoughts, that is your reality.

Remember my biking tour of Ireland? On my first day out there were a string of disasters that I won't bore you with but one episode was particularly meaningful for me. I was on a very narrow Irish country road with a huge ditch on the side and all I could think about was that I was going to fall into that ditch. I couldn't take my eyes off the ditch. The guide could see exactly what was going on and shouted "Look at the road, don't focus on the ditch!"

But it was too late for me. I was in the ditch. Fortunately, I was scraped up and scratched but nothing broke. What I learned was a valuable lesson: that my negative thoughts created my reality – literally.

Try to keep your focus on the positive. Keep your eye on the road that you want to follow, not on the obstacles, not on the pitfalls. How do you do that?

It starts with a daily practice of changing your mind by exercising your "**positive thought muscle.**" The way to do that is through **positive affirmations** that you repeat every day. It's like lifting small weights until those **positive repetitions become your thoughts** and you have a **strong spirit-lifting muscle**.

Louise Hay is the author of "*You Can Heal Your Life*," which is a classic book in the area of changing your thoughts to change your life. Here is what she says about positive affirmations:

> *Affirmations are like planting*
> *seeds in the ground. It takes*
> *some time to go from a seed to a*
> *full-grown plant. And so it is*
> *with affirmations – it takes some*
> *time from the first declaration to*
> *the final demonstration. So be*
> *patient.*

Whatever you think of menopause will shape your experience of menopause. Here is a positive affirmation that you can recite every day to help change how you think about yourself at this stage in your life:

> *I {your name} am a wise and beautiful goddess,*
> *Vibrating with life,*
> *Embracing my power,*
> *Speaking my truth, and*
> *Bursting with creative energy.*

Saying your name is important. If you can say this out loud, do it. And if you can say it while moving your body that is even better. Here's what I suggest:

Affirmation Exercise

- Bring your hands together over your head with straight arms, look up at your joined hands and say "I {your name} am a wise and beautiful goddess."

- Bring your hands down in a prayer position at your heart and say "vibrating with life."

- With your hands still in prayer position, bend at the waist and say "embracing my power."

- Reach down and grasp the back of your ankles or calves and say "speaking my truth."

- Stand up straight, sweeping your arms up in a V over your shoulders and say "bursting with creative energy."

- Repeat 7 times.

Try to recite your affirmation every day for the next three months and see what wonders develop in your life. Focus on your road ahead, your goal. Don't end up in the ditch like I did.

Recipe: Avocado Dip

- 1 large peeled and stoned avocado
- 2/3 cup regular or goat-milk plain yogurt
- 1 tomato, diced
- Dash or two of cayenne pepper
- Sea salt
- Fresh black pepper

Mash avocado roughly with a fork. Add yogurt, tomato and cayenne. Blend until smooth in a food processor, blender, or with a fork. Add sea salt and fresh black pepper.

Serve promptly with mixed raw vegetables.

Recipe: Arugula and Lentil Salad

- 1 cup dried lentils

- 1 teaspoon Dijon mustard
- ¼ cup extra virgin olive oil
- ¼ cup fresh lemon juice
- ½ teaspoon salt
- Freshly ground black pepper, to taste
- 2 garlic cloves mashed

- ½ cup Italian parsley, chopped
- 1 bunch (or bag) of arugula
- 2 cups cherry tomatoes
- ¼ pound feta cheese

Cook lentils according to package directions.

In small bowl, whisk together the mustard, olive oil, lemon juice, garlic, salt and pepper. Toss with the cooked lentils. This may be chilled for 3 hours and up to 24 hours.

Just before serving, add parsley, arugula, cherry tomatoes and feta. Adjust salt and pepper if needed.

Serves 6.

Chapter 3

The Energy Drain

Do you have the sense that you're dragging?

Many women in menopause or peri-menopause feel the loss of their energy. There are two main reasons that you may not be feeling as energetic as you once did.

The first is that your energy is being siphoned off. Do you remember the days of gas rationing when you had to line up at the gas station every other day depending on whether the last digit of your license plate was odd or even? In those days, people were going around sucking the fuel out of gas tanks. Well, that could be happening to you right now.

Who is sucking the energy out of you? Actual people or your internal critic or your own negative thoughts could be sapping your energy.

We talked in Chapter 2 about positive affirmations which go a long way to turning around the energy drain so that whatever energy you have is available to you for the purposes you have in mind.

Your Metabolic Fire

The second reason your energy may be down is that you haven't given your body the fuel that it needs to do all of the things that you want or need to do every day.

Your metabolism is the energy efficiency of your body in using the fuel that it has. And that fuel, of course, is the food that you feed yourself every day.

It's helpful to think about your metabolism as an old-fashioned fire in your wood-burning fireplace. What's the secret to a good blazing, long burning fire? It's the fuel. You can get heat and light from your fire if you give it a constant supply of twigs and paper but you better not stray too far from the hearth. If you leave to go to the store or run some errands, when you come back, that fire will have gone out.

Your fire needs big dry logs to keep going for a long time. If you're feeding your fire with twigs and kindling, you will be tending that fire all day long and you won't have the time - or the energy - to do all of the other things on your agenda because your flame will have burned out.

Your metabolism needs a good steady fuel source to burn long, strong and bright. And although there is lots of good press for lean protein and whole grains, the best fuel for that steady burn is fat! People are always shocked to hear that because we have become a nation indoctrinated in the **religion of low fat**.

Here is how each type of food you eat acts as a fuel for your metabolism:

- Fat – big, dry hardwood logs
- Protein – good solid logs
- Whole vegetables, fruits and grains – good steady fuel (artificial logs)
- Processed carbohydrates - kindling
- Processed sugars – twigs
- Alcohol – lighter fluid

What you never hear though is that fat is the preferred fuel for the body and it's what gives us a long steady source of energy. Fat is the equivalent of a good solid log for your metabolic fire.

In addition, fat gives us a feeling of satisfaction that is calming and puts lots of our late night snacking and cravings to rest.

The second most efficient fuel source is high quality protein. Protein can come from animal sources, like meat, fish and dairy, or vegetarian sources like beans, nuts and seeds.

Another good source of fuel is carbohydrates – fruits, vegetables and whole grains. They will also give you a long-lasting source of energy but only if they are in the whole, unprocessed form. If you're feeding your fire with processed carbs like bread, crackers, cereals, flavored yogurts, energy bars and frozen dinners, it's like throwing kindling on your fire. You get a boost but it doesn't last long.

One of the least efficient types of fuel is sugar and it's the one that we grab for most often when we feel our fire is low. In the afternoon we grab for a candy bar or energy bar, or Cokes and lattes to keep us awake and get through to dinner. The problem is that sugar burns out as fast as throwing paper on your fire.

Finally, keep in mind that alcohol is even worse than sugar and is like hosing your fire down with lighter fluid. It's very disruptive to the metabolic balance and leaves you feeling really drained after it takes you to great energetic heights.

So think about your metabolism as a fire and tend your fire wisely and you won't have to tend it constantly during the day.

You shouldn't have to be feeding your fire six times a day. This is what many people call **grazing**. If you're grazing, chances are you are eating low-fat snacks that don't hold you for more than 2 hours and so you have to eat again.

But if you eat a meal with healthy fats, that meal should burn bright for four or even five hours. That's important for people who are dieting because for some of us it's hard to *stop* eating once we start.

For some of us, it's also hard to control portions, so those 6 "mini" meals may not be so mini and can add up to much more than three normal meals.

Healthy Fats for Menopause

There are many benefits to eating high quality fats during menopause. But remember that not all oils and fats are created equal.

Heavily processed, hydrogenated, "trans" fats and oils that are used in prepared, packaged foods can be extremely damaging to your body.

But fats and oils from whole foods and other high-quality sources can steady your metabolism, keep hormone levels even, nourish your skin, hair and nails, and provide lubrication to keep the body functioning fluidly.

Our bodies also need fat for insulation and to protect and hold our organs in place.

Signs of insufficient high-quality fats are brittle hair and nails, dry skin, hunger after meals and feeling cold.

A healthy percentage of high-quality fat in a meal satisfies us and leaves us feeling full of energy, fulfillment and warmth.

On the other hand, when there are excess fats and oils in your diet, especially heavily processed fats, symptoms can include weight gain, skin breakouts, high blood pressure, liver strain and an overall feeling of mental, physical and emotional heaviness or sluggishness.

Fats: the Good, the Bad and the UGLY

There are good and bad fats and we need to spend some time figuring out which are which. So let's get to it.

There are many sources of healthy fats and oils. Remember that we want to focus on whole foods and so fat should be found naturally in our food such as in meats, especially organ meats, eggs and dairy.

Other healthy fats are found in whole nuts and seeds, and in their butters like almond butter or tahini (ground sesame seeds).

Whole foods such as avocados, olives and coconuts are great sources of healthy fat, along with wild salmon and omega-3 organic eggs. Experiment with these healthy fat sources and see which work best for you and leave you satisfied.

For sautéing and baking, try butter, ghee (clarified butter) or coconut oil because they don't break down when used for cooking at high temperatures. When sautéing foods at moderate temperatures, try organic extra virgin olive oil.

When it comes to oils, some are very good and others you should avoid. Oils like flaxseed, sesame, toasted sesame, and walnut oils are best used unheated in sauces or dressings on top of salads, veggies or grains.

Look for "organic," "first pressed," "cold-pressed," "extra-virgin," and "unrefined" on the labels.

Avoid the bad oils. What should you buy? When selecting oils, buy the highest-quality organic products you can afford, since cooking oils are the backbone of so many dishes.

Avoid all oils labeled "vegetable," "corn," "canola," "soybean," or "sunflower." Small amounts of safflower oil may be acceptable but not for cooking.

Words to avoid on the label are "expeller-pressed," "refined," "solvent extracted," and "polyunsaturated."

In summary, most people, especially infants and growing children, benefit from *more* fat in their diet rather than less.

But fats must always be high quality: avoid all processed foods containing newfangled hydrogenated fats and polyunsaturated oils.

Throw away all the corn oil, vegetable oil and Crisco in your pantry.

Instead, use only traditional vegetable oils like extra virgin olive oil and small amounts of unrefined flax seed oil. Use coconut oil for baking, and use animal fats (lard and butter) for occasional frying.

Eat foods high in fat such as egg yolks and other animal fats found in meats such as liver, and roasts or steaks with fat. Don't buy skinless chicken. It's much tastier cooked with the skin on.

Finally, use as much good quality butter as you like, with the happy assurance that it is a wholesome—indeed, an essential—food for you and your whole family.

10 Healthy Reasons to Enjoy Real Butter

Butter has gotten a bad rap for many years, starting in the last century with the rise of margarine, which we now recognize as a deadly trans fat. More recently, butter has been shunned in favor of olive oil and canola oil. But here's why we should reserve a place at the table for good old-fashioned butter.

A study from Lund University in Sweden shows that butter leads to considerably less elevation of fats in the blood after a meal compared with olive oil, flaxseed oil or a new type of canola oil. High blood fat normally raises cholesterol levels in the blood, which according to the discredited "lipid hypothesis," elevates the risk of atherosclerosis and heart attack.

Why doesn't butter raise blood lipid levels?

Researchers pointed out that 20 percent of the fat in butter consists of short and medium-length fatty acids. These are used directly as energy and do not stay around long enough to affect blood fat levels very much.

The researchers opined that although butter raises blood cholesterol in the long term, its short-term effects may actually be advantageous.

Not everyone agrees that butter's advantage over olive, canola or vegetable oils is only a short term phenomenon. Sally Fallon of **The Weston A. Price Foundation** is a staunch and eloquent advocate of the benefits of butter and disagrees that butter or cholesterol is a factor in the increase of cardiovascular disease.

The vast fat-free conspiracy

Since the early 1920's butter has been pushed aside in favor of margarine and other fad fats and vilified as a deadly saturated fat that causes heart disease. Yet for thousands of years before that, butter was a dietary staple of many cultures with no evidence of adverse health effects.

Between 1920 and 1960, Americans' use of butter declined from 18 pounds per person per year to 4 pounds, yet heart disease went from a relatively unknown condition to the number one killer. So how likely is it that butter is killing us?

According to Fallon, butter is the victim of a "vast fat-free conspiracy," formed by those who benefit from replacing healthy butter with disease promoting mass produced vegetable oils and trans fats.

The truth is that butter is good for you. Here are 10 benefits of eating real, fresh creamery butter:

1. Butter is the most easily absorbable source of **vitamin A** which supports the thyroid and adrenal glands, and in turn, the cardiovascular system.

2. Butter doesn't lead to excess body fat since its **short and medium chain fatty acids** are burned for quick energy and not stored, and it also gives a feeling of satiety that may decrease cravings and prevent over-eating.

3. Butter is rich in **anti-oxidants** including vitamins A and E, as well as selenium, protecting against heart disease as well as cancer.

4. Butter is a good source of **dietary cholesterol** which acts as an anti-oxidant, repairing damage from free radicals caused by rancid fats, vegetable oils and trans fats. Cholesterol is also important for the development of the brain and nervous system in children.

5. The saturated fat in butter consists of short and medium chain fatty acids which have **anti-tumor properties** and also strengthen the immune system.

6. Butter contains **conjugated linoleic acids (CLA)** which are cancer protective.

7. When in its raw state and not pasteurized, butter has an anti-stiffness property called the

Wulzen factor, that protects against arthritis, cataracts and hardening of the arteries.

8. Butter is a good source of **iodine** in a highly absorbable form and necessary for proper thyroid function.

9. It promotes **gastrointestinal health** and decreases rates of diarrhea in children.

10. Butter is a good source of **vitamin K2** which prevents tooth decay and builds strong teeth and bones.

Remember that the richest benefits are found in raw butter made from pastured cows. Look for "grass-fed" or "pastured" on the label.

Recipe: Northern Italian Quinoa Salad

- 1 cup quinoa
- ½ teaspoon sea salt
- ¼ cup extra virgin olive oil
- ¼ cup lemon juice
- 1 cup finely chopped red, yellow or green bell pepper
- ¾ cup finely chopped red onion
- ½ cup finely chopped cooked marinated artichoke hearts
- ¼ cup capers
- ½ cup currants
- ½ cup finely chopped fresh Italian flat leaf parsley

Cook quinoa according to package directions, let cool. Combine olive oil and lemon juice. Add peppers, onion, artichoke hearts, capers, currants and parsley, and toss. Add the quinoa and stir gently to combine. Salt and pepper to taste. Serve over mixed greens.

Recipe: Root Vegetable Soup

- 4 cloves garlic chopped
- 1 yellow onion chopped
- 1 tablespoon olive oil
- 2 carrots
- 1 turnip
- 1 rutabaga
- 1 parsnip
- 1 potato
- 1 sweet potato
- 1 can cannellini beans, rinsed and drained (optional)
- 2 quarts low sodium vegetable stock
- ½ teaspoon each of dried oregano, thyme and rosemary
- ½ teaspoon salt
- ½ teaspoon red pepper flakes

Sauté onion and garlic in olive oil in a large soup pot over medium heat until softened. Add salt and red pepper flakes.

Peel and chop remaining vegetables and add to the pot with the vegetable stock and herbs. Cook on low heat until vegetables are soft. Add additional liquid if needed.

Add beans, if desired, and cook for 20 minutes more.

Puree soup with blender or immersion blender if desired.

Adjust salt and pepper to taste.

Chapter 4

Lose Weight by Breaking All the Diet Rules

Our weight is mostly determined by our lifestyle and diet, but there is also an element of personal preference. Do we think that the Calista Flockart silhouette is attractive or do we prefer a more substantial Oprah look.

What Is A Healthy Weight?

It's important to be realistic about our weight as we get a little older. Annemarie Colbin, a whole foods chef and founder of the Natural Gourmet Institute, likes to remind women of two things. One is that nature makes us bigger as we get older and it's a good thing because it comes at a time of life where we feel free to "throw our weight around."

The other reason is that as our ovaries stop producing estrogen, body fat is actually an estrogen producing organ that takes up the slack. You want some estrogen but not too much. Likewise, you want some body fat but just not too much.

What is Your Body Type?

It's important to keep in mind the idea of bio-individuality that we talked about before. We are all unique and that is certainly true when it comes to our body composition. Women often make themselves crazy by comparing themselves to unrealistic (and often unnatural) body images that we see in TV, movies and magazines. When we are determining the right weight for our bodies, it's not helpful to compare a woman of wisdom and substance with a starlet.

Even among women of the same age there are vastly different body types. You were born with a body type and you are not going to be able to alter your build no matter what. So it is helpful to get clear on what your body type is so you can be realistic about how much you can change.

Ayurvedic Body Types

In Ayurvedic medicine, the ancient healing art of India, there are three body types, Vata (Winter), Pitta (Summer) and Kapha (Spring). These correspond roughly to the three body types you might have heard of: Ectomorph, Endomorph and Mesomorph.

Vata (Winter) embodies the qualities of cold, dry air. These types are the contemporary idea of beauty: thin-boned, tall and skinny (the supermodel) or short, slim and petite. They have sharp minds and a tendency to worry, are light sleepers and have nervous dispositions. Vatas usually have a fast metabolism, difficulty gaining weight, and weak intestines so they often don't absorb their nutrients very well.

Pittas (Summer) embody the qualities of fire. These people are more physically oriented, with more muscle and a fiery temperament. They usually have yellow or reddish colored skin that is sensitive to rashes. They often sweat profusely and are easily irritated but have a strong athletic constitution. They are well-organized, intelligent and charismatic; emotional, competitive and passionate. Pittas need a good 8 hours of sleep. They have enormous appetites for food and life experience and can become gluttons if not careful.

Kaphas (Spring) embody the wet, heavy characteristics of Spring. They are generally big-boned, full-bodied, and physically strong, and they tend to gain weight. They have strong skeletons that protect them from osteoporosis. Their skin is often pale and cool and their eyes are often large and dark.

Kaphas are easygoing, slow, methodical types with balanced, peaceful temperaments. They radiate confidence even when quiet or shy. They have a slow metabolism, strong intestines and easily absorb nutrients so they can eat less. Their main health risks are obesity and heart disease.

Ayurveda is a very complex way of viewing the body, health and nutrition, and even the entire universe. The very simple idea that you can glean from this little introduction is that bodies are different with different strengths, weaknesses and metabolisms.

If you are interested in pursuing the ideas of Ayurveda, try reading Dr. John Douillard's "The 3-Season Diet" to learn more.

When is Your Weight a Health Concern?

Abdominal Fat

Some weight gain at midlife is innocuous. Remember that weight gain in perimenopause may go away when you reach menopause as your metabolism adjusts and stabilizes.

But some weight gain is a health risk. Excess belly fat is more dangerous than fat on your hips or thighs. Beware of the apple-shaped figure more than the pear-shaped body.

Abdominal fat contributes to insulin resistance, wreaking havoc with your blood sugar levels.

It also can produce excess androgens (male hormones) and estrogen which is associated with increased risk of heart disease, breast cancer, uterine cancer, diabetes, kidney stones, hypertension, arthritis, incontinence, polycystic ovary disease, urinary stress incontinence, gallstones, stroke and sleep apnea.

Waist/hip ratio is a measure of the health risk of excess weight. Here is how to gauge your waist/hip ratio:

> With a tape-measure, measure around the fullest part of your buttocks, and then around the narrowest part of your torso.
>
> Divide your waist measurement by your hip measurement.
>
> A healthy ratio is less than 0.80. The ideal ratio is 0.74. If you are above 0.85 you have increased risk of all of those conditions.

What is Your Body Mass Index?

Another way to determine whether your weight puts you at a health risk is to calculate your body mass index.

Here is the formula:

> Divide your weight in pounds by your height in inches squared. Multiply that product by 703.

If your BMI is less than 18.5 you are underweight. From 18.5 to 24.9 is normal; 25 to 29.9 is overweight; and 30 or more is obese.

Just reducing your BMI by 1.0 can dramatically improve your health, lower blood pressure and balance hormone levels.

Women who gain 20 pounds in their adult years are said to have a decline in vitality and physical function equivalent to smoking. But losing just 5 or 10 pounds makes a great improvement.

Why do we gain weight in menopause?

Metabolic Slow Down

According to Dr. Christiane Northrup, our metabolism slows down from 10-15% around menopause. If you continue to eat the way you always have, there is a good chance that you will gain weight during perimenopause. But remember, some of that weight gain will be temporary and many of us lose it and settle back to our normal weight after menopause.

Toxic Weight Gain

Dr. Pamela Peek in her book "Fight Fat After Forty," talks about abdominal weight gain in menopausal women arising from "toxic stress."

Toxic stress is common at this stage of life and comes from resurfacing of childhood traumas, perfectionism, relationship challenges (divorce and caregiving), job stress, acute or chronic illness, and even dieting.

Late afternoon and evening eating may be triggered because at this time of day hormones that help battle stress (serotonin and cortisol) are at a low point and make us more vulnerable to emotions. That can make us more likely to grab for refined carbohydrates and sugary snacks to bring us back to normal.

Lack of Estrogen

It's essential that every menopausal woman understands the sad case of the fat rats as told by Gary Taubes in his book "Why We Get Fat And What to Do About It."

A researcher at the University of Massachusetts in the 1970s did some experiments with rats to determine the relationship between estrogen, weight and appetite.

In his first experiment, he removed the ovaries from rats and they became ravenous, ate voraciously and quickly became obese.

In his second experiment, he removed the rats' ovaries, but put the poor rats on a strict diet. What do you think happened? They still got obese even though their calories were restricted to a level where they should not have gained weight. But these rats also became completely sedentary, lacking energy and only moving to get food.

The rats became gluttons, but if they couldn't eat more, they conserved their energy and moved less i.e., lost energy and became lazy.

In his third experiment, the researcher removed the ovaries but gave the rats estrogen injections. The result: the rats did not overeat, did not become lazy and did not become obese. They were perfectly normal.

So that is how it is with rats deprived of estrogen. Why does that happen?

On a biochemical level, estrogen interferes with an enzyme called lipoprotein lipase (LPL). LPL pulls fat from the blood stream into fat cells for storage. When estrogen is high, LPL can't pull fat into the cells. But once estrogen is gone, LPL goes to work packing fat into the cells.

Now the rats (and the theory goes, menopausal women), eat voraciously because all their fuel is going into storage in the fat cells and isn't available for the rest of the body. The fat cells are hogging all the calories.

So with estrogen lower at menopause, is there another way to slow down the LPL packing fat into our cells?

There is. LPL is controlled by insulin, the primary regulator of fat metabolism. Insulin is a concern for everyone, not just diabetics.

The more insulin we secrete the more active LPL will be at packing those fat cells.

Insulin also slows down the LPL action on the muscle cells so that fat energy doesn't get in to fuel our muscles. Insulin diverts all fat to storage mode and not to energy expenditure.

It gets worse. Not only does insulin signal LPL to pack fat into your cells, it also suppresses another enzyme inside the fat cells called hormone-sensitive lipase (HSL).

HSL is our friend. It breaks down the fats in our cells and releases them into the blood stream making us leaner. But insulin stops HSL from breaking down fat so it keeps it trapped in our bodies.

Insulin increases the fat we store and decreases the fat we burn.

What to do? We have to control insulin to restore a healthy regulation of our fat cells.

What else does this research show?

Calories do not matter.

These rats become obese not because they eat too much but because they eat *at all*. Every calorie goes to stored fat.

We don't get fat because we eat too much. We eat because we are getting fat. It is like children in growth spurts. They don't shoot up because they are eating so much. Their bodies tell them to eat because they are growing.

Marathoners are not lean because they run so much, they run so much because they are lean and have the energy to run. If our fat metabolism is not functioning correctly and we cut calories, we simply stop moving. We start conserving energy.

Researchers are now thinking about this type of fat as a tumor. The tumor is growing and requires more energy to sustain itself.

So it doesn't help to count calories. Besides, they are notoriously inexact. When it comes to calorie counts on restaurant menus and frozen entrees at your supermarket, don't believe everything you read.

A recent study found that calories on the labels of packaged foods could be understated by anywhere from 18% to 200%.

The study from the Friedman School of Nutrition Science and Policy at Tufts University examined the calorie content of 18 side dishes and entrees from national sit-down chain restaurants, 11 side dishes and entrees from national fast food restaurants, and 10 frozen meals purchased from supermarkets in the Boston area. It concentrated on choices advertised as having low calorie content or less than 500 calories.

Researchers found that the information provided by restaurants on menus or websites understated the actual calorie content measured by an average of 18% and that in two instances by almost 200%. They also found that free side-dishes offered with a meal can exceed the calorie count of the main entrée.

The frozen entrée manufacturers did a little better, underestimating their calorie content by only 8% on average. Publishing their results in the Journal of the

American Dietetic Association, the researchers pointed out that the better performance by manufacturers may be attributed to the fact that the FDA monitors packaged nutrition fact panel labels more strictly than restaurant disclosures.

Another possible cause of the inaccuracy of the restaurant chain information is a discrepancy between the portion size contemplated by the disclosure information and the actual portion set before the diner.

The authors also pointed out that the wrong calorie information can contribute to weight gain since a 5% increase in daily calorie intake would translate to a 10 pound gain over a one year period.

These results underline the futility of state and local government efforts to legislate our every calorie in an effort to trim our collective waistlines. Calories make sense for some people but counting them day in and day out is not a successful strategy for most. In the long run it's just not practical.

What's a dieter to do? Learn portion control rather than calorie counting. Order baked, steamed or broiled rather than fried anything. If you do check calories, assume that the count is overstated by 20% and eat accordingly.

Even better: cook at home.

In another study, career dieticians were asked to calculate the number of calories in a meal. Could they do it? No. They were hundreds of calories off.

That makes a big difference. If we eat 20 calories extra a day (would you even know?) starting in your 20's you would be obese by your fifties.

So what is the answer? It's controlling your insulin.

The low carbohydrate diet

How insulin works.

When you eat carbohydrates, your body converts the carbohydrates into glucose, which is a sugar, and sends it into the blood stream. Your body can use only a limited amount of glucose at a time and then it has to clear the glucose out.

It does this through the pancreas which excretes the hormone insulin. The insulin signals the cells to open up and take in sugar.

When the cells are full, the insulin signals the liver to send the rest of the glucose into storage as fat.

While the body is in this fat storage mode, it can't burn any fat. It can't multi-task. It's one thing or the other.

The 4 Stages of Feeding and Fat Burning

Your body has 4 feeding stages:

- Fed (0-3 hours after eating),
- Early Fasting (3-18 hours after eating),
- Fasting (18-48 hours after eating) and
- Prolonged Fasting (48 + hours).

If you graze and eat small meals every 3 hours or so, you are in a constant fed state, which is the fat storage mode, all day long.

In the early fasting state, the liver manufactures glucose from stored glycogen, protein and stored fat. During this stage, you are actually releasing fat from your stores.

On a higher fat, lower carbohydrate diet you can go longer without eating because the fat makes you feel more satisfied for longer periods of time, so you stay in the early fasting, fat-burning mode.

Here is the best fat-burning strategy:

- Eat 2 or 3 satisfying meals a day to maximize the time in fat burning mode.
- Don't eat less than 3 hours before going to bed.

That's it! Just give it a try.

Sugar and Processed Foods

The first step in a low-carbohydrate diet is to get rid of added sugars. These include:

- white or brown sugar
- honey
- molasses
- maple syrup
- corn syrup
- fruit juices

It also includes any of the following listed on food packages:

- sucrose
- dextrose
- fructose
- maltose (beer)
- lactose
- glucose
- agave nectar
- high fructose corn syrup
- brown rice syrup
- evaporated cane juice
- fruit juice concentrate
- corn sweetener

The second step is to get rid of all processed carbohydrates. This includes bread, breakfast cereals, crackers, cakes, cookies, instant oatmeal, bagels, pasta, pretzels and chips.

A good rule of thumb is to avoid anything in a package that has more than three ingredients.

Good Carbohydrates

Grains are what we think of when we think of carbohydrates but carbs also include fruits and vegetables.

Whole Grains. The most important thing to do for weight loss in menopause is to make the change from processed to whole carbohydrates. Whole grains are found as close to nature as possible, with minimal processing or additives.

They include whole oats which are whole groats, or steel cut or rolled oats, but not instant oatmeal in a package or oatmeal bread or oatmeal cookies.

Whole wheat. The whole grain form of wheat is the wheat berry which has the bran and fiber intact. It is found in whole wheat or whole grain bread. But be careful. Although bread and crackers and wraps can be made with whole grains, the whole grains are then processed to be of little benefit to us.

Brown rice. Make the switch from white rice to brown. It would take about 8 bowls of white rice to get the nutrients of one bowl of brown rice.

Quinoa, millet, barley, and kasha are also good choices when it comes to whole grains and it's worth experimenting with them.

Grains are best eaten earlier in the day for weight loss, and better avoided for dinner.

Vegetables. Whole vegetables are good for weight loss but if you are particularly sensitive to insulin, you should know that some vegetables are higher than others in carbohydrates.

Leafy greens and salads are low in carbohydrates while beans, carrots, parsnips, corn, peas, potatoes and sweet potatoes (the starchy vegetables) are highest in carbs.

Dark Leafy Greens

The standard American diet is lacking is so many ways, but perhaps the greatest deficiency is in dark, leafy green vegetables.

Greens have a broad range of impressive nutritional benefits. They contain vitamins A, C, E and K as well as prodigious amounts of calcium, iron, potassium, magnesium, phosphorous and zinc, not to mention, the fiber, folic acid, chlorophyll, micronutrients and phytochemicals that protect against disease. They are also rich in cancer fighting antioxidants. Generally speaking, the darker the leaves, the more nutrient dense is the vegetable.

When I talk about dark, leafy greens, I am not talking about iceberg lettuce or Boston bibb or even romaine, although they all have a place at the table. I mean serious greens like kale, bok choy, collards, Swiss chard, mustard greens, broccoli rabe, escarole and dandelion.

These greens are powerful allies for your body, assisting in purifying the blood, strengthening the immune system, promoting good intestinal bacteria and improving circulation, liver and kidney function.

If you're already eating some broccoli and spinach and mixed green salads, good for you. But now it's time to upgrade your choices and expand your nutritional horizons.

Take some extra time and really explore the produce section of your market. Once a week pick a green you've never tried before, take it home (after you pay for it) and find a simple recipe.

Experiment. Don't give up after one try. Give greens a chance. Then a second chance. And a third chance.

Still hesitating? Start with kale. It's a member of the cabbage family and comes in a variety of shapes and sizes, including curly leafed, red and dinosaur (a choice that will fascinate the kids). Its health benefits are legion and studies have associated diets high in cruciferous vegetables such as kale with a lower incidence of many cancers, including lung, colon, breast, ovarian and bladder cancers.

Besides leafy greens, the second best choices for a low carbohydrate diet include asparagus, broccoli, Brussels sprouts, cauliflower, celery, eggplant, green beans, leeks, mushrooms, onions, peppers, snow peas, sugar snap peas, summer squash, tomatoes and zucchini.

Fruit. Fruit is great and full of fiber and antioxidants. But for weight loss fruit should not be considered a "free food."

Fructose is the sugar found in fruit and the liver converts fructose into fat more rapidly than any other sugar (sucrose, lactose or glucose).

Excess fructose can lead to fatty liver disease and cirrhosis just like excess alcohol. Although the fructose in natural fruit is not as bad as high fructose corn syrup and other processed fructose sweeteners, it can be a problem for those with insulin resistance, metabolic syndrome, diabetes, high blood pressure or high cholesterol.

According to Dr. Joseph Mercola, for those with a sensitivity and anyone interested in weight loss, it is important to limit fructose from fruit to 15 grams per day. Here are some sample numbers.

Fruit	Serving Size	Grams Fructose
Cantaloupe	1/8 melon	2.8
Raspberries	1 cup	3.0
Blackberries	1 cup	3.5
Cherries	10	3.8
Strawberries	1 cup	3.8
Pineapple	1 slice	4.0
Grapefruit	½ medium	4.3
Nectarine	1 medium	5.4
Peach	1 medium	5.9
Navel orange	1 medium	6.1
Banana	1 medium	7.1
Blueberries	1 cup	7.4
Apple	1 medium	9.5
Watermelon	1/16 melon	11.3
Pear	1 medium	11.8
Raisins	¼ cup	12.3
Grapes	1 cup	12.4
Apricots, dried	1 cup	16.4
Figs, dried	1 cup	23.0

Importance of Protein at Midlife

Beef, pork, ham (unglazed), bacon, lamb, veal or other meats are generally high in protein. All meats should ideally be grass-fed, pastured, organic, and free of antibiotics and growth hormones. Remember that all-natural on the label does not guarantee anything.

Processed meats (sausage, pepperoni, hotdogs) should have a carbohydrate content of about 1 gram per serving. These should also be from grass-fed animals and in addition to the requirements for meat, should be nitrate and nitrite free.

Poultry (chicken, turkey, duck or other fowl) should also be free-range, cage-free or pastured, and should say vegetarian feed, no antibiotics or hormones. The issue of growth hormones and menopausal women is important – we don't need to be ingesting growth hormones at this time in our lives.

How to Read Labels on Meat

The most important thing to remember in purchasing meat is to avoid products from cruel confined animal feeding operations (CAFOs) or factory farms. According to the documentary "King Corn," a hundred years ago all cattle were fed a grass diet and allowed to graze on open land. In the film, agriculture professor Allen Trenkle of Iowa State University states that today up to 90% of feed for cattle consists of corn, a diet that will kill the cattle within 6 months unless they are dosed with antibiotics.

In CAFOs cattle are confined in a small space so that they won't be able to move or expend any calories, and they are fed continually. The result is that they can be sold to packing plants in 4 to 5 months as compared to 2 years for grass fed animals. Not a happy life for the animals and not a good choice for the consumer.

The result of feeding cattle in this manner is an obese animal whose muscle tissue looks more like fat. That's according to Dr. Loren Cordain of the University of Colorado, and author of "The Paleo Diet," who was interviewed for the film. In fact, he says, a T-bone steak produced in this way contains about 9 grams of saturated fat compared to 1.3 grams in a grass fed animal. As for ground beef, he says it is "really fat disguised as meat" with 65% of its calories coming from fat.

To avoid meat from factory farms, ideally you would purchase beef and dairy from a local farm that you know, where animals have been humanely raised, grass fed, pastured and not administered antibiotics or added hormones.

To find a farm or a store in your area selling products from grass fed pastured animals, visit Eat Well Guide (www.EatWellGuide.org) and search for the type of product you are looking for. There are also internet sources if nothing is available in your geographic area.

In your market or at a farmer's market, check the labels on beef and dairy products for the following:

> ***Organic*** – The "USDA Organic" seal means that the product, the producer and the farmer all meet the USDA's organic standards and have been certified by the agency. For beef and dairy, this means that animals have been provided outdoor access and pasture, that they have not used antibiotics or hormones and have been fed 100% organic feed without animal by-products.
>
> ***Antibiotics*** – Animals that have not been given antibiotics during their lifetimes can be labeled "no antibiotics administered," "raised without antibiotics" or "antibiotic-free."
>
> ***Grass-Fed*** – This label means an animal was fed grass rather than grain but not necessarily for its entire life. Some may have been "grain-finished" meaning that they were fed grain from a feedlot prior to being slaughtered.
>
> ***100% Vegetarian Diet*** – If raised on a diet of grain, usually corn, this label ensures that the animals were not also fed animal by-products.
>
> ***Hormones*** – Animals raised without added growth hormones can be labeled

"no added hormones" or "no hormones administered," but the USDA has prohibited the use of the term "hormone free."

Natural – This is not a meaningful label. USDA guidelines state that "natural" meat products can undergo minimal processing and cannot contain artificial colors, artificial flavors, preservatives or other artificial ingredients. However, it does not assure that the animals are organic, humanely raised or free of hormones or antibiotics.

Pasture Raised – This indicates that the animal was raised on a pasture and ate grasses, rather than being fed grain in a feedlot. It is similar to "grass fed" but indicates more clearly that the animal was actually raised outdoors.

It takes some extra time, effort and money to find responsible sources for meat products, but the benefits to small farms and to your own health are well worth it.

Fish and shellfish are also good protein choices and include tuna, salmon (wild caught only, not farm raised), flounder, bass, trout, shrimp, scallops, crab and lobster.

Whole eggs are another healthy protein choice but look for eggs from cage-free chickens or pastured chickens allowed to roam, and only fed a vegetarian diet.

Limit your dairy products to cheese, cottage cheese and cream from grass-fed cows and it should be preferably raw. This includes cheeses made from raw milk.

Other good protein sources are nuts and seeds.

Tips for Additional Weight Loss

If you are not losing weight making these basic changes to your diet it may be that you are more insulin resistant and need to cut back on carbo-hydrates even further.

Most low-carbohydrate diets recommend a minimum of 72 carbohydrates per day. However, it depends on your body. You might be able to lose weight on 200 carbs per day while someone else would have to restrict their carbohydrates even more dramatically to begin to lose weight.

If you are not losing, the next step would be to cut back or cut out grains altogether and see what happens. Grain-free diets (like the Paleo Diet) are becoming more popular for this reason.

Also for weight loss, you should avoid milk and yogurt because the lactose sugar may impact your insulin production.

Cheeses should be limited to 4 ounces per day of high quality (not processed or fake) cheese and cream should be limited to 4 tablespoons per day.

Still no weight loss? Try cutting back or cutting out fruit.

If that doesn't work your next step might be to cut back or cut out starchy vegetables.

You may have to cut carbohydrates down to as little as 0 – 20 grams per day to lose weight if you are particularly sensitive to carbohydrates.

Remember you are not cutting calories. You should not be hungry. You may still be on a 2,000 calorie diet (but who's counting?) because you will be eating more protein and fats to make up for the difference and avoid hunger.

You have to find the level of carbohydrates that your body can tolerate without storing fat.

It is best to reduce your carbohydrates slowly since you may actually feel worse in the first few days from withdrawal from the sugars in the carbs.

If you find that you need to follow a very low carbohydrate diet, try the Atkins Diet or the Duke University Medical Center "No Sugar, No Starch" Diet as summarized in Gary Taubes book "Why We Get Fat." However, don't forget the quality of your food is important. Atkins allows fake nutrition bars twice a day and Duke has no requirements for food quality.

Exercise – Strength Training

According to Pamela Peeke, women who do not strength train lose about 7 pounds of muscle every 10 years and that equates to a reduction in metabolism of about 350 calories per day. This does not happen to women who lift weights.

Between the ages of 30 and 80, you can lose as much as 60 percent of the strength in your back, arm and leg muscles.

We lose muscle mass at the rate of 4% per decade from 25 to 50 and then 10% per decade after that.

Weight training is important to do at least twice a week. So go to the gym, get a personal trainer or do it at home.

Dr. Peeke has an easy guide to weight training that you can do in your own home with just hand weights in her book "Fight Fat After Forty."

Weight Loss Plan at Midlife

Here is your basic midlife weight loss plan:

- Cut out all added sugars and processed carbohydrates.

- Eat only whole unprocessed grains and whole natural vegetables.

- Don't eat carbohydrates (grains, legumes, vegetables or fruit) alone. They should always be paired with healthy fats.

- Grains, beans, legumes and starchy vegetables should be grouped together and should be limited to no more than 2 servings per day and preferably not at dinner.

- Fruits should be limited to no more than 2 servings per day or 15 grams of fructose.

If you are particularly sensitive to sugar, try modifying the basic rules for the **Carbohydrate Sensitive Plan**:

- Cut back or cut out all grains including bread, and even whole grains.
- Cut back or cut out all beans, legumes and starchy vegetables.
- Cut back or cut out fruit.

And if that doesn't work you may be highly sensitive and need to modify the basic plan for **Highly Sensitive Plan**:

- Cut all carbohydrates from all sources to 20 grams per day, limited primarily to leafy greens and non-starchy vegetables.

- Remember bio-individuality. You want to reduce your carbohydrate intake gradually to find the level where you are losing weight but also are feeling good, with lots of energy.

Recipe: Vegetable Spring Rolls with Szechuan Peanut Sauce

- 1 cup freshly ground organic peanut butter
- ¼ cup low sodium organic soy sauce
- ¼ cup organic Asian sesame oil
- 3 tablespoons unseasoned rice vinegar
- 2 tablespoons finely chopped garlic
- 2 tablespoons grated peeled fresh ginger root
- 1 ½ teaspoons Asian chili paste (or 1 tsp. dried hot red pepper flakes)
- 1 tablespoon hoisin sauce
- 1 ½ to 2 tablespoons fresh lime juice
- ¾ cup coconut water (or plain water)

In a blender or food processor or by hand, blend all ingredients (with salt to taste) until smooth. Transfer sauce to a jar with a tight-fitting lid to keep, covered and chilled, up to 1 week. Makes about 2½ cups.

- Rice Spring Roll Wrappers

- Red cabbage, finely chopped
- Napa cabbage, finely chopped
- Carrots, grated
- Broccoli Sprouts

Soak spring roll wrappers in warm water and dry in accordance with package directions.

Place grated vegetables and sprouts in the middle of the wrapper and add 1 tablespoon of sauce. Fold bottom of wrap over filling, fold in sides totally covering the filling, then roll neatly.

Serve with additional sauce on the side for dipping.

Recipe: Beef and Arugula Stir-Fry

- ½ pound sirloin, cut into strips
- 2 tsp olive oil
- 1 TB minced fresh ginger
- 1 clove garlic
- 2 red bell peppers cut into very thin strips
- 1 to 2 bunches washed arugula
- 2 tsp kuzu
- 2 tsp tamari
- 2 tsp apple cider vinegar
- 1/4 cup water

Stir-fry the beef in a pan with 2 tsp of oil over medium-high heat for about 2 minutes or until browned. Remove beef and set aside.

In the same pan, in remaining oil, stir-fry ginger and garlic for 2-3 minutes and then add the bell pepper. Cook for another 2-3 minutes.

Mix together fresh arugula and bell pepper mixture in a serving bowl.

In a small bowl, combine kuzu, tamari, vinegar and water.

Place kuzu mixture into skillet and cook over medium heat until sauce starts to thicken. Return beef to skillet and cook for 1 minute, just enough to warm up beef.

Add the beef to the serving bowl with the arugula and bell peppers. Mix and serve warm.

(From *Integrative Nutrition* by Joshua Rosenthal)

Chapter 5

Energy and Mood Swings

When we talk about our moods we are talking in part about the quality and quantity of our energy. Is our energy high and positive so that we have a good, happy, optimistic outlook and we're moved to action and getting things accomplished? Or is it low and negative so that we're flirting with depression?

There are other variations on the quality and quantity of our energy. Is it high and negative so that we're jittery, fearful and anxious? Or is it low and positive so that we are calm, restful and maybe even meditative?

OUR ENERGY STATES	
HIGH AND NEGATIVE Jittery, Fearful and Anxious	HIGH AND POSITIVE Happy, Optimistic, Productive
LOW AND NEGATIVE Sad, Depression	LOW AND POSITIVE Calm, Restful, Meditative

Sometimes we have a rather narrow view of energy and its function in our lives. We think about it as something that we use to enable us to "do things" or move our bodies, whether it's walking the dog, playing tennis, driving kids all over the map, working out at the gym and even just sitting quietly.

But what we often fail to realize is that not only do we **USE** energy, but *WE ARE ENERGY*. In fact, that's ALL we are. We are nothing but energy.

We tend to think of ourselves as solid, massive bodies made of bone and muscle, organs, tissue, skin and hair. But if you know anything about physics you know that's only part of the picture.

For example, we go about our lives thinking that things like the chair you are sitting on is solid. But in fact, at a more basic level that chair is almost all space. It's a collection of atoms - little electrons zooming and circulating around a nucleus. But mostly that chair consists of the space around those particles and not the particles themselves. That empty space is more than 90% of the whole thing. What holds the chair together is the energy that's generated by all of that action of zooming and spinning. It holds those particles in a form that we experience as a chair.

The same goes for each of us. We appear to be solid bodies but we are really vibrating, pulsating, electric power plants. We are pure energy.

Test Your Energy

Let's do a little exercise. I want you to get comfortable with thinking about yourself as pure energy. So plant your feet flat on the floor, close your eyes, take a deep breath, and let it out. Relax your hands in your lap or wherever it feels most natural and comfortable. Take a deep breath, relax your shoulders, and let it out. Relax any tight spots in your body. Take another deep breath, and let it out. Now, just feel your body as energy, feel yourself as a power generator.

So what's your energy like? Does that experience make you want to go to sleep? Is it uncomfortable for you to be still like that? Can you feel yourself pulsating and vibrating with life? Are you a pulsating power house or a faint ember?

We often have the idea that how we feel and what our energy level is has to do with what is going on in our lives and things that have happened to us, how much sleep we got and the people we have to deal with. But a lot of how you feel will actually depend on what fuel you are burning and that fuel is the food you eat.

You've heard this before but it bears repeating. We are what we eat. The food we take into our mouths goes into our stomachs, where it gets digested and eventually assimilated into the bloodstream. Our blood is what creates our cells, our organs, our skin, our hair, our brains and even our thoughts and our feelings. We are the walking totality of what we eat.

When you eat food with more energy, you will have more energy. Everything we put in our mouths has its own unique energy, beyond vitamins, minerals, fats and carbohydrates. When we eat we assimilate not only the nutrients, but also the energy of the food.

Ani Phyo, a raw foods expert, has said "*Food is the most intimate thing you can buy...Unlike clothes and shoes that dress the outside, food goes into your body and builds who you become.*"

When we eat food we take in its distinct qualities and energetic properties, depending on where, when and how it grows, as well as how it is prepared. By understanding the energy of food, we can choose meals that will create the energy we are seeking in our lives.

You never really hear about the concept of food having energy, but it makes sense. Vegetables have a lighter energy than proteins. Meat from tortured animals raised in confined animal feed lots (CAFOs) or factory farms, has a different energy than fish caught in the wild.

Plants sprout from seeds. Some animals hatch from eggs. Others are birthed by their mothers and are nurtured through infancy. Each of these things has a different energy.

Even among different vegetables, there are different types of energy. Consider how particular plants grow. Leafy greens, such as spinach, kale, dandelions, collards, Swiss chard and bok choy, grow by reaching up toward the sky. They soak in the energy of the sun and generate chlorophyll.

When we eat foods rich in chlorophyll, we take in the sun's energy as well as oxygen for our blood. For this reason, greens are powerful mood enhancers, lifting the spirit and lightening our mood when we feel tense. They give us upbeat energy. This is important for midlife women who are at risk for depression and often feel their mood is low.

Squash, pumpkins and other gourds grow at ground level and help balance moods and energy levels, keeping them steady.

Root vegetables, such as onions, potatoes, sweet potatoes, carrots, turnips, parsnips, rutabagas, beets and burdock root, grow deep into the ground. They grow slowly and absorb the nutrients from the soil in which they grow. Therefore, they have a strong downward energy and provide heartier more sustainable energy. They are great for grounding us when we feel unfocused, nervous, anxious, stressed or over-stimulated.

On the other hand, processed foods like donuts, candy bars, protein bars and diet sodas are as dead as they possibly can be. They have been stripped of all nutrients and anything that could possibly spoil or go rancid. Then they are packed with sugar. We grab for these products as a "quick energy fix." However, there is no energy in those dead processed sugary foods and within an hour you will still need real energy.

The Power of Root Vegetables

Consider what kind of energy you get from a donut. How would that differ from the energy you get from eating organic roasted root vegetables?

I have experienced firsthand what a difference eating different vegetables can make in my energy levels. I have a habit of eating root vegetables whenever I have a big meeting or presentation to ground me and keep me focused.

But the real power of root vegetables was proven to me by a friend's daughter who was in high school. Melanie was active in theater and had been performing before audiences since she was 3 years old when she began to give piano concerts. Then, all of sudden in her first year of high school, she developed paralyzing stage fright. Her voice and music coaches didn't know what to do. Her parents wanted to take her to a psychiatrist or put her on prescription beta blockers or anti-anxiety medication.

What was really going on with Melanie? Her mother said that she had recently become a vegetarian like many teen-aged girls who refuse to eat anything with a face. So what was she eating? In the morning she usually ran out of the house with a glass of orange juice and a cereal breakfast bar. For lunch she packed a peanut butter and jelly sandwich on whole grain bread. For dinner she would have pasta and maybe some salad.

Melanie had fallen into the same trap as many girls who become vegetarians: she hardly ever ate an actual vegetable and she was eating lots of processed carbs. Her next performance was in three days.

I asked her mother to make a big pot of root vegetable soup with onions, garlic, vegetable stock, carrots, potatoes, sweet potatoes, turnips, parsnips, rutabagas, beets, and anything else she could find that grew underground, and feed it to Melanie for the next three days. Melanie's stage fright disappeared and she gave a fabulous performance.

Whenever Melanie had a performance after that she asked "Mom, where's my soup? Did you make my soup?" She hasn't had stage fright since. That is the power of the right food at the right time.

What happened with Melanie was that she was full of nervous energy and she needed to calm down, get grounded and steady herself. The root vegetables do that for her and they can work the same way for women in menopause who often report feelings of anxiety.

The diet Melanie was eating, breakfast bars, bread for lunch and pasta for dinner, was a very high carbohydrate diet which may not have been a problem for her except that it also featured mostly refined carbohydrates and that means a high sugar diet.

Imagine how you might feel if you stayed away from processed carbohydrates and found vegetables and grains that are as close as possible to their natural unprocessed state.

Great Grains

Whole grains are an excellent source of nutrition, because they contain essential enzymes, iron, dietary fiber, vitamin E and B-complex vitamins. But most importantly, from an energy point of view, because the body absorbs grains slowly, they provide sustained and high-quality energy.

When they have not been processed they keep all the components of their original, natural state: fiber, vitamins and minerals. Processing removes these elements. So remember almost all breads and cereals, cold or cooked, are processed.

Always look for the whole grain in its natural state. Some good choices are:

- Brown rice
- Buckwheat (kasha)
- Oats (whole groats or steel cut)
- Barley (hulled)
- Polenta
- Millet
- Quinoa
- Wheatberries
- Wild rice

And grains can be very convenient because you can cook a big batch and then freeze the leftovers or just store them in the refrigerator for use the same week.

Here is a little summary chart that comes in handy to show which foods can lead to different types of energy.

Energy Quality	Food
Grounded Relaxed	Root vegetables Sweet vegetables Millet, brown rice Meat, Fish High Quality Fats Beans
Light Creative Flexible	Leafy Greens Wheat, barley, quinoa Fruit Raw foods Chocolate
Tense Anxious	Sugar Refined carbohydrates Caffeine Nut Butters Alcohol

Why Do We Have Mood Swings and Depression at Menopause?

When we reach peri-menopause and menopause, our estrogen levels begin to fluctuate and they can fluctuate wildly.

Estrogen inhibits certain hormones in the brain so when we have low estrogen, estrogen no longer inhibits that hormone and the imbalance in the brain can lead to depression.

But when estrogen swings the other way and we have an excess, it throws our levels of copper and zinc out of whack and this leads to exaggerated stress reactions, serious mood swings and also depression. We can't deal with stress.

Either way, too little or too much estrogen puts you at risk of depression. But diet can help.

The Link Between Dieting and Depression

How many women do you know who are on a diet? How many women do you know who are on anti-depressants? Is there a link?

Julia Ross, a clinical psychologist and author of *The Mood Cure: The 4-Step Program to Take Charge of*

Your Emotions- Today!, sees a connection between skyrocketing rates of depression and the diet obsession.

She notes that statistics show that we are **100 times more depressed** than we were in 1900 and that fully **50% of Americans over the age of 14** are experiencing "significant debilitating depression and/or anxiety." That is shocking.

At the same time, she says, our diets have deteriorated to the point of "epidemic malnutrition." She notes that in 1965, after the processed food industry had been going strong for about 10 years, the average U.S. woman was deficient in 3 nutrients. By 1990 that deficiency had risen to 13 nutrients.

Ross traces the problem in part to a beauty infatuation starting in the 1960's that led women to slash fat and calories from their diets.

Compounding the problem, she says, was the introduction in the 1970s of highly addictive corn syrup sweeteners that are twice as sweet as sucrose and twice as addictive.

This combination led to women wanting to starve themselves for the Twiggy look but being unable to resist hi-carb processed foods that made them fat.

Ross, an expert on the treatment of eating disorders and addictions, says the first symptoms of mal-nutrition are emotional; what she calls "false moods."

She categorizes four false moods depending on which of 4 neurotransmitters (serotonin, catecholamines, GABA and endorphins) are not being produced by the brain because of the absence of certain amino acids in the diet. Amino acids are the building blocks of proteins and that's where we get them in our diets.

It's estimated that 86% of Americans have low levels of neurotransmitters.

Some people lacking the proper neurotransmitters become irritable or quick to anger, sometimes even becoming violent, which she believes leads to many incidents of domestic violence.

Other people exhibit signs of depression, becoming apathetic or having no energy, suffering shakiness, teariness and generally an increased inability to deal with stress. Still others are overwhelmed by anxiety.

How do you avoid falling into the trap of these false moods? Ross advises a whole foods diet that sustains stable blood sugar for the longest time possible. This includes saturated fats, high protein and fresh vegetables and after that, whole carbohydrates as tolerated.

Ross claims that diet is essential to correcting neurotransmitter deficiencies and mood disorders, and that the single most important nutrient required is **protein** because the brain is "protein dependent."

Many menopausal women today are trying to eliminate or cut back on animal protein, but fail to find a replacement protein source and rely instead on increasing carbohydrates.

Ross states that everyone needs at least 25 to 30 grams of protein ***per meal*** as compared to 18 to 20 grams per meal recommended by many diets. The USDA recommends only about 56 grams ***per day*** for men and *46 grams per day for women*.

Here is a chart with the various amounts of protein that you can get from common foods.

Food	*Quantity*	*Protein (grams)*
Beans	1 cup	15
Cheese, firm	1 ounce	6-10
Cheese, soft	1 ounce	2-4
Cottage cheese	1 cup	30
Eggs	1	6
Meat, poultry, fish	3-3 ½ ounces	17-27
Milk	1 cup	8-10
Nuts	¼ cup	2-7
Oatmeal, cooked	1 cup	6
Peanut butter	2 tablespoons	8
Rice, cooked	1 cup	6
Ricotta cheese	1 cup	28
Seeds	1 ounce	6
Yogurt	1 cup	8-10
Greek Yogurt	6 ounces	13-18

Good Sources of Mood-Boosting Protein

Protein comes in many different forms. Most people think of protein as animal products like steak, chicken, turkey, fish, lamb and pork, as well as dairy products like milk, yogurt and cheese.

But protein is also contained in vegetarian sources like beans, grains, nuts and seeds. Each of those sources will provide a different type of energy.

When it comes to eating animal protein, look for products that are of the highest quality, organic, free of antibiotics, grass-fed and humanely treated. If the animal was healthy and happy and had good energy, then you will be healthy and happy and get good energy from it.

Joshua Rosenthal in his book, *Integrative Nutrition: Feed Your Hunger for Health & Happiness*, suggests that different types of meat will give you different types of energy. For example, if you eat too much cattle, you may find that you have taken on the energy of a cow. Not an attractive image. Now think about the cow compared to a chicken. If you eat too much chicken, you may get an overabundance of nervous, twitchy energy. Now think about fish, gliding swiftly through water, going with the flow. You can come up with your own examples and it's an interesting theory.

How Much Protein Do You Need?

We all know that protein is good for us and in fact it's one of three necessary macronutrients along with carbohydrates and fat. But can you get too much of this good thing?

Gout has long been known to be associated with greater intakes of animal protein which is high in uric acid.

According to Paul Pitchford in his book, Healing with Whole Foods, diets high in protein carry other proven health risks, among them osteoporosis and kidney disease.

Dr. Andrew Weil agrees that too much protein puts a strain on the digestive system and can damage both the kidneys and the liver.

Dr. T. Colin Campbell, author of *The China Study*, believes that an excess of protein is associated with any of 18 or more chronic degenerative diseases, including cancer.

That's why it's important to evaluate the amount of protein you're getting in your diet. You could also be getting too little. If so, you could be feeling spacey, jittery, fatigued, and weak. You could also lose weight, lose healthy color in your face, suffer anemia, or see unwanted changes in your hair color and texture.

On the other hand, if you're getting too much protein, you could have low energy, constipation, dehydration, lethargy, or weight gain. You might have a heavy feeling, sweet cravings, "tight" or stiff joints, or halitosis. You could also shows signs of osteoporosis since an excess of animal protein can leach calcium from your bones.

As a general rule, Americans eat too much protein. But it's not uncommon for menopausal women and young girls to get too little protein. Everyone's needs are different and you need to experiment and find the level that gives you optimum energy and lifts your mood.

The recommended daily allowance (RDA) for protein as determined by the U.S. Department of Agriculture is .8 grams per ideal weight in kilograms. That comes out to about an average of 56 grams per day for men and 46 grams per day for women. When measuring your food, that translates to one or two servings of animal protein per day.

Dr. Weil believes that there is a growing consensus that the proper range of protein in the diet is 10 to 20 percent of calories consumed. On a 2,000 calorie diet, this translates to between 200 and 400 calories.

In addition, he advises to choose from protein sources that are less concentrated than animal sources such as beans, whole grains and vegetables which have the added benefits of fiber, carbohydrates, healthy fats and phytonutrients that protect against diseases.

Your Gut Health and Depression

One particular neurotransmitter is associated with symptoms of depression and that is the "feel-good neurotransmitter" serotonin. When we think of depression we think of something out of balance in our brain but really over 90% of the serotonin in your body is located in your gut.

In fact, the gut is often referred to as "the second brain." Our nine-meter long gut is lined with over 100 million neurons – more brain cells than we have in our spinal cord.

Our gut is also home to over 100 trillion bacteria which help us digest food and absorb nutrients.

Studies have repeatedly shown that a healthy gut reinforces a positive outlook and behavior, while depression and a variety of behavioral problems have been linked to an imbalance or lack of gut bacteria.

So it's important to maintain a healthy balance of good and bad gut bacteria.

How does that balance get out of whack?

One way is eating too much sugar and processed foods which feed yeast and fungal growth at the expense of healthy bacteria.

Another problem is taking antibiotics which kill bacteria indiscriminately, both good and bad. If you have taken a course of antibiotics, your gut could be low on the good bacteria we need for our immune system and so much more.

In order to restore your gut bacteria balance, it's important to eat probiotics.

Natural food sources of probiotics include:

- Yogurt
- Sauerkraut
- Pickles and pickled vegetables
- Kimchi, fermented Korean cabbage
- Sour dough bread
- Kombucha (fermented green or black tea)
- Soy sauce
- Tempeh, a fermented food usually made from soybeans but also from other beans or grains
- Kefir, a fermented dairy drink similar to yogurt

Foods to Put You in a Bad Mood

While protein is the number one food that you need to avoid depression and improve mood, and probiotics help keep your gut healthy, there are a number of foods that promote bad moods in us.

Sugar

The number one bad mood food is sugar, either in its pure form, or as part of refined carbohydrates containing white flour. Taken together they have drug-like mood-altering powers.

These foods force your brain to release natural feel-good neurotransmitters – serotonin and endorphin – disrupting brain chemistry and leading to the need for more of these neurotransmitters to boost mood again, and the cycle just continues.

Another effect of these foods is that they raise your insulin levels very quickly and then blood sugar levels drop precipitously. That's when you become hypoglycemic and get grouchy, headachy or weepy. Those bad moods are completely food triggered.

Gluten

The second bad mood food is gluten. Although whole grains can be a great addition to your diet, some people are sensitive to the gluten contained in wheat, rye and barley.

Gluten sensitivity can result in bloating, digestive distress, bowel problems, diabetes and higher colon cancer risk.

Gluten can irritate, inflame and rupture the lining of the digestive tract to the point where nutrients are not getting absorbed by your body. And if nutrients necessary for regulating mood are not being absorbed you can suffer headaches, depression and manic-depression.

Wheat grown in the U.S. today is a hybrid developed to increase its gluten content to make breads and pastries puffier. But it also makes the flour much more difficult to digest.

This new gluten has been called a "brain allergen" and acts like an opiate. That's why you may feel that you love your bread or pasta and feel comforted by it. If you think you are addicted to bread, you may very well be.

Gluten affects many sensitive people by making them feel lethargic, unfocused and exhausted. If these are your symptoms, you may want to get tested for gluten sensitivity or do an elimination diet to see if your symptoms resolve if these are removed from your diet.

Vegetable Oils

The third bad mood food category is vegetable oils. We already talked about eliminating these from our diets. These are all vegetable oils (except olive oil) including corn, soy, canola, sunflower, safflower, peanut, sesame, walnut, etc.

Vegetable oils are pressed out of seeds, nuts and beans that are high in Omega-6 fats. These Omega-6 fats are essential to clot blood, shed the lining of the uterus when we menstruate, constrict blood vessels, and produce inflammation to kill viruses and bacteria.

But consuming too many Omega-6 fats results in inflammation all over the body - including the brain.

Omega-3 fats are also essential to build the walls of our brain cells. If we don't get enough Omega-3s though, Omega-6 steps in with its inflammation producing properties.

The result is that our inflamed brain stops sending and receiving signals, and this leads to depression. It's very interesting that increased rates of depression over the last hundred years track very closely with the increased rates of vegetable oils in our food supply.

Aspartame

The fourth mood destroying food is aspartame contained in the artificial sweetener NutraSweet and in many diets foods, especially sodas. It can cause headache, bloating but also mood disturbances such as depression, irritability, confusion, anxiety attacks, insomnia and phobias. This is because it inhibits serotonin.

Just like sugar, it can raise levels of insulin and has actually been linked to diabetes. And it can also be highly addictive.

Caffeine

Another mood altering food is caffeine. This can also inhibit the brain's level of the anti-depressant serotonin and also the body's sleep-inducing melatonin. Caffeine also depletes the body of mood enhancing nutrients like the B vitamins, vitamin C, potassium, calcium and zinc. It takes only a small amount – 2 small cups a day or one large mug.

MSG

Finally, all chemical additives and artificial colorings or flavorings in processed foods can adversely affect your mood but one of the biggest offenders is MSG – monosodium glutamate, which is well known to trigger depression. It's important to recognize this on labels because it goes by many aliases.

The following ingredients on a label always indicate the presence of MSG:

- Glutamate
- Monosodium glutamate
- Monopotassium glutamate
- Glutamic acid
- Yeast extract
- Hydrolyzed protein
- Calcium caseinate
- Sodium caseinate
- Yeast food
- Hydrolyzed corn gluten
- Gelatin
- Textured protein
- Yeast nutrient
- Autolyzed yeast
- Natrium glutamate

The following foods often contain MSG or create MSG in the course of processing:

- Carageenan
- Natural pork, beef or chicken flavoring
- Bouillon, broth, stock
- Whey protein concentrate
- Whey protein
- Whey protein isolate
- Flavor(s) or flavoring(s)

- Maltodextrin
- Citric acid
- Ultra-pasteurized products
- Barley malt
- Pectin
- Protease
- Protease enzymes
- Anything enzyme modified
- Enzymes anything
- Malt extract
- Malt flavoring
- Soy protein isolate
- Soy protein concentrate
- Anything protein fortified
- Anything fermented
- Seasonings

Primary Foods™ and the Meaning of Your Life

Primary Foods™ is a concept created by Joshua Rosenthal in his Integrative Nutrition™ program. It teaches that all we typically consider as nutrition is really just a secondary source of energy.

The fun, excitement and love of daily life have the power to feed us so the food we consume becomes secondary. This is especially true when we're children or we're deeply in love, or working passionately on a project.

But think about when you are depressed, which is a common complaint in menopause. You may actually be starving for primary food. No amount of secondary food will do. You can eat as much as you want but you never feel satisfied. We often look into the refrigerator for something to eat, when all we really want is a hug or someone to talk to. Sometimes when we are craving a food, what we really need to do is tend to our primary foods.

Primary foods feed you, but they don't come on a plate. They are things like a meaningful spiritual practice, an inspiring career or other work, regular and enjoyable physical activity, and honest and open relationships that feed your soul and your hunger for living. All of these constitute primary food.

At midlife, changing hormones change the way we view life. From the time we were little girls, estrogen has been circulating in our bodies and even at a young age, the estrogen builds our brain centers for observation, communication, gut feeling or "female" intuition and caring. These are all the things that make us the women we are.

According to Dr. Louann Brizendine, author of *The Female Brain,* when a woman is pregnant, she produces much more estrogen as well as progesterone, which has a calming effect. And when she gives birth, a mother is flooded with oxytocin, the maternal bonding hormone that makes her nurturing. "The mommy brain" makes women committed to care giving and putting the needs of the family first.

But Dr. Brizendine explains that at menopause the "mommy brain unplugs," and snaps the circuits that make women great communicators and emotional beings. Women lose some of their drive to care and tend for others, and to avoid conflict at all costs.

With lower levels of estrogen, progesterone and oxytocin, women begin to be more self-centered and shift from care-giving mode to a focus on their own personal development. This is what Christiane Northrup refers to as "the lifting of the estrogen veil."

Because of this fundamental shift, menopause is a natural time to examine your life and what you want to accomplish for yourself. A good way to do that is to examine your primary foods of spirituality, physical exercise, career and relationships.

Understanding the changes on your body can help relieve much of the anxiety and guilt women feel at menopause. Focusing on your own personal development does not mean that you are abandoning your family. The best thing that women in menopause can do for those they love, is to love themselves.

Recipe: Scrambled Eggs and Spinach

- 4 eggs
- 2 tablespoons butter
- 1 leek thinly sliced
- 2 carrots finely chopped
- 1 cup coarsely chopped watercress (or spinach)
- 1 tsp Tabasco sauce
- 1 tsp turmeric
- unrefined sea salt and pepper to taste

Beat eggs with turmeric, Tabasco, salt and pepper. Heat 1 tablespoon butter in skillet, and cook leeks and carrots until softened (about 10 minutes). Remove to a plate.

Add 1 tablespoon of butter to skillet, scramble eggs until just cooked. Add leeks, carrots and watercress.

Recipe: Quinoa Tabouleh

- 1 cup quinoa
- 2 1/4 cups water
- 1 cucumber, seeded and diced
- 1 tomato, seeded and diced
- 1 bunch mint, minced
- 1/2 bunch parsley, minced
- 2 tablespoons lemon juice
- 3 tablespoons extra virgin olive oil
- unrefined sea salt to taste

Rinse quinoa thoroughly and add to boiling water with pinch of salt. Reduce to low and simmer for 20 minutes. Fluff with fork and let sit 10 minutes.

Combine all ingredients in a large bowl and mix gently. Adjust seasonings if necessary.

Chapter 6

Hot Flashes and Night Sweats

What are hot flashes?

You may know this common symptom of menopause all too well. But many women in the early stages of perimenopause don't figure out what is going on.

When I was still working as a lawyer in my early forties, I noticed a very strange thing happening. Every morning rushing out to work, I would get in my car, drive past the first traffic light on my route and inevitably get stuck in traffic at the second light. As I sat there I could feel the heat rise from my chest to my face and head, and feel tightness all along my scalp. All of sudden no matter how cold it was outside, I was opening the window for a breeze. This happened just about every day but it wasn't until years later that I realized I was having my first hot flashes.

If you haven't had the pleasure yet, a hot flash is a momentary sensation of heat that may be accompanied by sweating. Some people also refer to it as a "hot flush" when that heat and sweating is accompanied by a red, flushed look in the face and neck.

When your hot flash occurs at night, it's referred to as night sweats and can interfere with sleep, compounding your problems.

For some women, hot flashes and night sweats can also be accompanied by rapid heart rate which they can even describe as an anxiety attack. Some believe that they are having symptoms of heart disease. I heard Oprah once tell her audience about having heart palpitations and going to a series of heart specialists, none of whom could find anything wrong with her. Later, while interviewing a menopause expert, she realized for the first time that she did not have a heart condition but she was having a form of a hot flash.

It makes you wonder how many women are put on anti-anxiety medications because of their heart palpitations when they are really just having a power surge.

The severity and duration of hot flashes vary among different women. They can last for a minute or for an hour. When they are finished some women experience chills.

You might experience hot flashes for a brief time during menopause whereas others have them for the rest of their lives, although generally they become less severe as time goes by.

Although we think of hot flashes as a necessary evil that inevitably accompanies menopause, it's not quite the universal experience that many of us think it is.

According to Dr. John Lee, author of *What Your Doctor May Not Tell You About Menopause: The Breakthrough Book on Natural Hormone Balance*, only about 50% of women in the United States experience hot flashes, and only about 15% seek medical advice for their symptoms. While that rate is comparable to other industrialized countries, it is much higher than in less developed countries where menopause symptoms are rare.

Menopause symptoms are usually blamed on dropping estrogen levels. But women in less developed countries experience the same physical drop in estrogen levels yet don't suffer the symptoms. Even in the U.S., all women suffer the same drop in estrogen but not everyone has to frantically peel off their clothes several times a day.

Why do we get hot flashes and night sweats?

What is going on in our bodies physiologically when we start to feel the heat mounting? Actually, it is not completely understood. We do know that the blood vessels near the surface of our skin dilate. But what causes that?

Dr. Lee explains that in our reproductive years levels of progesterone and estrogen naturally drop during our cycle. When that happens our hypothalamus in the brain signals our pituitary gland to tell our ovaries to start producing more hormones. But when we get to menopause, our ovaries don't respond to that signal anymore. The hypothalamus doesn't understand why the ovaries aren't paying attention and, as Dr. Lee says, it starts "shouting." It gets so loud, it's like waking up the neighbors. The signals start affecting a neighboring part of the brain that controls capillary dilation and sweating. Voila, you have a hot flash because your progesterone and estrogen levels are low and your ovaries don't respond anymore.

Common Sense Relief for Hot Flashes

Tearing off your clothes is one way to help relieve your symptoms. It does help and there are other very practical common sense things that you can do to relieve your symptoms. Here are some suggestions:

- The most important thing is to stay cool. That means wearing light layers of breathable fibers like cotton and open neck shirts, and putting your turtleneck sweaters away for a while.
- Use ceiling fans, open the windows and put your air-conditioning on in April, if you have to, in order to get a good night's sleep.
- Putting a drop of peppermint essential oil on the back of your neck can also cool a hot flash.
- Put ice on your wrists, or a cool compress on your forehead or chest.
- Use natural fibers like cotton for sheets and nightwear.

- Keep a bottle of ice water handy and sip on it to cool yourself down when a flash starts, night or day.
- Keep a spray bottle of cool water on your nightstand to spritz yourself when needed.
- Eat cooling foods that you would find in the summer like salads and melons. Take an ice pack to bed and put it on your chest when you feel a flash coming on.

You also want to be aware of certain foods and activities that will bring on your hot flashes and try to minimize your triggers. Some typical triggers include:

- Stressful situations
- Tight clothing
- Heat
- Cigarette smoke
- Foods such as caffeine, alcohol, sugar and spicy dishes

Balancing Estrogen and Progesterone

While we may think that the problem is low estrogen, the truth is that at menopause, our estrogen only drops 40 to 60%. Our progesterone levels, however, can drop to zero. So although it might look like the problem is low estrogen, it is more likely low progesterone.

In menopause, in order to achieve hormonal balance, it's important for most women to increase their progesterone levels and/or decrease their estrogen levels. Even if hormone levels are lower, as long as progesterone and estrogen still maintain their balance, we may avoid symptoms.

In Chapter 7, we'll talk about supporting the adrenal glands with a whole food diet to help produce more progesterone. That's one way to restore balance.

On the other side of the equation is reducing the amount of estrogen in our bodies. There are two ways to do that naturally. One way is through phytochemicals found in plant foods and the other is by boosting our fiber intake.

Balancing Hormones with Phytochemicals

Let's talk about phytochemicals first. "Phyto" means plant and phytochemicals are just natural compounds found in plants. The two primary phytochemicals that we are concerned with at menopause are phytoestrogens and bioflavonoids.

Phytoestrogens are plant compounds that have estrogen-like properties. They are not human estrogen but they act like estrogen in the body. They are considerably weaker than the estrogen produced by your body and they compete for the same receptors on your cells.

Almost every cell in your body has estrogen receptors. If you take in lots of weak phytoestrogens, they take up space on the receptors. This blocks stronger estrogens and can help if your body has excess estrogen. If you have low estrogen, they will contribute a small amount of estrogen to boost your levels.

Phytoestrogens are found in more than 300 plants and the most common ones in our diets are apples, carrots, oats, plums, olives, potatoes, tea, coffee and sunflower seeds.

Phytoestrogens are also strong antioxidants so they prevent free radical damage which contributes to that look of aging that we start to notice around menopause. They can help us look younger.

Bioflavonoids are another type of phytochemical found in herbs and fruits that help reduce estrogen. These are plant chemicals that also compete with excess estrogen for receptor sites. Some good sources are cherries, cranberries, blueberries, bilberries, grape skins and many whole grains.

Another way to keep estrogen levels down is by eating enough fiber. When your body is finished with estrogen, it goes to the liver and is dumped into the intestines to be excreted. If not excreted, it gets reabsorbed and recirculated in the body. But fiber binds to excess estrogen and helps the body eliminate it.

The best fiber for this job is soluble fiber found in apples, bananas, citrus fruits, strawberries and pears. Beans are also full of soluble fiber, especially kidney beans. Whole grains are also good sources of soluble fiber, with oats and barley being the best choices.

Is Soy a Menopause Health Food?

One food often recommended for menopausal women is soy. It's claimed to eliminate hot flashes, relieve PMS symptoms, migraines, prevent weight gain, decrease fat and increase lean muscle.

In 1999 the FDA approved a claim for soy as a health food that reduces the risk of coronary artery disease. The FDA has since admitted that its approval was a mistake.

There are many reasons to avoid soy altogether. According to Sally Fallon Morell of the Weston A. Price Foundation and many others, soy contains anti-nutrients and toxins that interfere with the absorption of vitamins and minerals.

Soy foods contain anti-nutritional factors such as saponins, soyatoxin, phytates, protease inhibitors, oxalates, goitrogens and estrogens. Some of these factors interfere with the enzymes you need to digest protein. While a small amount of anti-nutrients would not likely cause a problem, the amount of soy that many Americans are now eating is extremely high.

Soy also interferes with thyroid function which is already a problem for many menopausal women. This is because soy is a goitrogen - a substance that blocks the synthesis of thyroid hormones. It also interferes with iodine metabolism which is necessary for proper thyroid function.

Soy also contains phytates (phytic acid) which bind to metal ions, preventing the absorption of certain minerals, including calcium, magnesium, iron, and zinc -- all of which are necessary in your body. This is particularly problematic for vegetarians, because eating meat reduces the mineral-blocking effects of these phytates (so it is helpful—if you do eat soy— to also eat meat).

You may have heard that soy isoflavones are great for menopausal symptoms. These are a type of phytoestrogen, but the soy versions are known to disrupt endocrine function, may cause infertility, and may promote breast cancer in women.

Many people point to Asians and claim that they eat soy and have lower rates of cancer and heart disease as well as fewer symptoms of menopause. However, Asians actually eat very small amounts of soy compared to Americans. In this country, soy protein has made its way into over 2,700 fast foods and processed food products. In Asia on the other hand, soy is only eaten after it has been fermented to remove the anti-nutrients.

The only safe soy products to eat are fermented soy products. Examples of fermented soy include:

- **Tempeh** a fermented soybean cake with a firm texture and nutty, mushroom-like flavor.

- **Miso**, a fermented soybean paste with a salty, buttery texture (commonly used in miso soup).
- **Natto**, fermented soybeans with a sticky texture and strong, cheese-like flavor.
- **Soy sauce**, which is traditionally made by fermenting soybeans, salt and enzymes; be wary because many varieties on the market today are made artificially using a chemical process.

Tofu is not a fermented soy product and should be minimized or avoided.

The biggest objection to soy is the fact that over 90% of the soy crop grown in the U.S. is genetically modified so that it can resist the weed-killer RoundUp made by Monsanto. GMO soy is loaded with this toxic pesticide.

The plants also contain genes from bacteria that produce a protein that has never been part of the human food supply. There aren't many studies showing the effects of these proteins, so eating GMO soy is taking an unknown risk.

Recipe: Roast Turkey and Kale

- 1 tablespoon olive oil or butter
- 1 red onion cut in thin strips
- 1 bunch curly kale, cut in thin ribbons
- 1/2 pound roast turkey breast, cut into bite-sized chunks
- 1 tablespoon balsamic vinegar
- salt and pepper to taste

Saute onions in oil or butter over medium low heat for 15 minutes until lightly brown. Add kale and stir until wilted. Add turkey and cook until warm. Add balsamic vinegar, salt and pepper. Serves 4.

Recipe: Tahini Lemon Dressing

- 2 tablespoons tahini (ground sesame seeds)
- juice of one lemon
- 1/2 cup water
- 1 teaspoon of tamari soy sauce

Whisk ingredients together to combine. Serve over salad or fresh vegetables.

Chapter 7

Breast Health at Menopause

No discussion of menopause can ignore the threat of breast cancer. Since 1950, breast cancer has risen by 60 percent. In North America alone a woman dies of breast cancer every 12 minutes.

What's causing this? Experts agree that 80% of breast cancer is driven by diet and the environment. Only the other 20% is genetic. We can do something to change our diet and environment and in turn, our risk profile. Breast cancer is not all about your genes.

It is well known that estrogen is a major contributor to breast cancer as well as to endometrial cancer. In part, this is because estrogen encourages cell growth. Its job is to build up cells in the uterus in preparation for pregnancy. This build up continues on a monthly basis until progesterone kicks in to stop the growth and to begin the maturation process of cells.

One big factor in the rise in breast cancer rates is the use of synthetic hormone replacement therapy. Prescription HRT has been called the greatest experiment ever performed on women. It was prescribed for decades without clinical trials proving either its safety or efficacy.

Years after HRT became standard treatment for menopause, researchers finally decided to study its effects. The Women's Health Initiative was a huge study that found that ***women using PremPro, a synthetic form of progesterone, had a 29% higher rate of breast cancer.***

Dr. John Lee, in his book *What Your Doctor May Not Tell You About Menopause: The Breakthrough Book on Natural Hormone Balance*, attributes this high rate not to all hormone replacement therapy but to the high estrogen doses that have typically been prescribed, and to the synthetic progestin (e.g. Provera) that accompanies it.

According to Dr. Lee here are some of the factors contributing to breast cancer risk:

a.   Breast cancer is more likely to occur in premenopausal women with high estrogen levels and low progesterone levels.

b.   Pregnancy occurring before age 30 is known to have a protective effect because of the high levels of progesterone during the pregnancy.

c.   Women without children are at a higher risk.

d.   In addition to breast cancer, ovarian and endometrial cancers are more common in women who receive estrogen replacement therapy (without progesterone) or HRT which combines estrogen with synthetic progestin rather than natural progesterone.

It is essential to recognize that not all estrogens are created equal when it comes to their effect on the breasts. There are 3 types of estrogen, all competing for the same cell receptors:

    a. **Estradiol** has the most stimulating effect on breast tissue.
    b. **Estrone** is the second most stimulating.
    c. **Estriol** has the weakest effect on breast tissue.

Low levels of estriol relative to the other two forms correlate with increased risk of breast cancer, while higher levels of estriol correlate with remission of cancer.

And it's not just the absolute level of estrogen that causes a problem but whether it is balanced by progesterone. *Breast cancer is over 5 times more common in women with low progesterone than in women with normal progesterone levels.*

And this is true for other cancers as well. *Women with low progesterone have 10 times the risk of all malignant cancers.*

Breast Cancer and Diet

As mentioned before, 80% of breast cancer risk is attributable to diet and environment. Diet is a major factor in breast cancer as well as uterine cancer.

The problems with our diets are both quantity and quality.

Quantity is important because excess food leads to obesity and obesity leads to higher estrogen levels that feed cancer. Studies have shown that women who lose weight can reduce their risk of breast cancer. It's important to remember that body fat can actually be considered an estrogen generating organ.

In addition to the quantity of food, the quality is important. Research has shown that the typical Western diet which is high in poor quality fats – all those omega-6 fats - and high in poor quality meat, sugar and refined carbohydrates, but low in fruits, vegetables, whole grains, fish, nuts, seeds and fiber, contributes to high breast cancer risks.

Researchers at the Kimmel Cancer Center at Thomas Jefferson University wanted to test the theory that elevated fat levels found in a typical American-style diet play an important role in the growth and spread of breast cancer.

They fed laboratory mice the equivalent of a Western diet. Mice were placed on a diet that contained 21.2% fat which the researchers believed reflects a typical Western diet. A control group of mice was fed a diet of only 4.5% fat.

The mice were already predisposed to develop mammary tumors. But those who were fed the Western diet developed larger tumors that grew faster and metastasized more easily, compared to the animals eating a control diet. In fact ***with the Western diet, the number of tumors almost doubled, and they were 50% larger.***

The researchers noted that breast cancer rates are five times higher in Western countries than in other developed countries and people in countries with a low rate who later adopt a Western diet show an increased rate of the cancer. That means that diet has a significant effect on breast cancer development.

Avoiding the standard American diet is a first step toward reducing breast cancer risk. The same diet that we have been talking about to lose weight, lower estrogen, and improve mood will also reduce your risk of breast cancer.

Now let's look as some special foods that are particularly helpful in fighting cancer.

Phytoestrogens and Breast Cancer

We talked about phytoestrogens and how they are weak forms of plant estrogens. They can help reduce estrogen in our bodies if our levels are too high and increase estrogen if our levels are too low. This is a miraculous property of food that pharmaceuticals cannot replicate.

Flax Seeds

One particular class of phytoestrogen is lignans. Lignans also act as antioxidants. Dietary sources of lignans include seeds (sesame, sunflower and pumpkin), grains (rye, barley, wheat and oats), and broccoli and beans.

But the tiny *flax seed has over 800 times the amount of lignans* as any of the other dietary sources.

An ancient plant, flax (also known as linseed) goes back 5,000 years and Hippocrates recommended it in 650 B.C. for abdominal pain. Charlemagne was so taken with the special benefits of flax that in the 8th century he required by law that his subjects consume it.

When eaten, lignans are broken down by bacteria in the gut into 2 estrogen-like compounds that circulate through the liver. These compounds have been proven in animal studies to help prevent breast and colon cancer by preventing tumor growth.

In postmenopausal women, studies have shown that eating 25 grams (about four tablespoons) of ground flax seed a day changes the way estrogen is handled in the body and provides protection against breast cancer.

According to Christiane Northrup in her classic book, "*The Wisdom of Menopause*," flax seed lignans "help in both the prevention and treatment of breast and colon cancer because of their ability to modulate the production, availability, and action of the hormones produced in our bodies."

Sesame Seeds

Pumpkin seeds come from pumpkins, sunflower seeds come from sunflowers and sesame seeds come from... sesames?

Actually, sesame seeds come from a tropical plant called *Sesamum indicum* which is believed to have originated in Africa and today is commercially cultivated mostly in India, China and Mexico. In the Caribbean and southern U.S., sesame seeds are often known by their African name, *benne*.

Archeological evidence suggests that the sesame plant was grown at least 2,500 years ago and it has a rich mythological heritage. An Assyrian legend tells of the gods drinking a wine made from sesame seeds on the day before they created the world.

The seeds, which vary in color and can be black, white, yellow or red, grow in pods which burst open when ripe. This is said to be the basis of the magic phrase of "open sesame" in the Arabian Nights.

In cooking, sesame seeds are not just important as a decoration on Big Macs. For their diminutive size, they pack a potent array of nutrients. They are a good source of calcium, magnesium, manganese, phosphorous, vitamin B1 (thiamine) and zinc.

Sesame seeds are an excellent source of copper, an important mineral element in the body's anti-inflammatory systems which has been known to help reduce the pain and swelling associated with rheumatoid arthritis.

In addition, sesame seeds have been found to have the highest levels of phytosterols among the most common seeds and nuts in America. Phytosterols are plant compounds believed to reduce blood levels of cholesterol. Their cholesterol-lowering effect may be heightened by the presence of two lignans they contain called sesamin and sesamolin.

The seeds can be eaten whole, ground into a paste known as tahini or processed into an oil. They have a mild, nutty flavor and a slight crunch.

Cruciferous Vegetables

Another category of phytochemicals that are important for breast health are the cruciferous vegetables which are also known as the Brassica family. These are vegetables in the cabbage family like broccoli, cabbage, kale, cauliflower, Brussels sprouts, bok choy, collards, kohlrabi, mustard greens, rutabaga, turnips, and Chinese cabbage. Arugula, horse radish, radish, wasabi, and watercress are also in the same family.

These vegetables contain a special chemical called sulforaphane which improves the liver's ability to detoxify carcinogens and other toxins. It takes only 3 to 5 servings a week to get the health benefits.

But you have to be careful not to overcook cruciferous vegetables. This is because there is an enzyme called myrosinase in broccoli, for instance, that is necessary to form the sulphoraphane but cooking it too much will destroy the enzyme.

You also don't want to eat too much of these vegetables in the raw form because they are goitrogens. This means that they interfere with thyroid function and can promote a goiter, if they are not cooked. Ideally these vegetables should be steamed gently for two to four minutes to protect the myrosinase and to limit the goitrogenic effects.

Watercress

Long associated with tea sandwiches and white gloves, watercress contains a plant compound that may help fight breast cancer.

According to research conducted at the University of Southampton and published in the *British Journal of Nutrition and Biochemical Pharmacology*, the plant compound known as phenylethyl isothiocyanate, may suppress breast cancer cell development by 'turning off' a signal in the body which is necessary to cancer cell growth.

When cancerous tumors outgrow their blood supply, they send out signals to normal tissues to feed them oxygen and nutrients. The compound in watercress interferes with those signals resulting in the starvation of the cancerous growth by blocking essential blood and oxygen. Prior studies had found the same plant compound to be effective in blocking the growth of prostate and colon cancer cells.

In the study a small group of breast cancer survivors ate a bowl of watercress and then had their blood tested over the next 24 hours. The researchers found significant levels of the plant compound in the blood following the watercress meal, and the signaling function was also measurably affected in the blood cells of the women.

Watercress is a member of the cabbage or cruciferous family and although much more delicate than its relatives, kale, broccoli, mustard greens and collards, it offers many of the same health benefits including a wealth of antioxidants. It is an excellent source of calcium and is rich in iron, zinc, potassium and magnesium. It also provides vitamins C, A, E and K as well as the B vitamins, including folate.

Watercress has been recommended to insure eye health because it contains a rich supply of two carotenoids, lutein and zeaxanthin which protect against cataracts. In herbal practices it is used to help to normalize cholesterol and blood pressure, and as a blood cleanser and breath freshener.

It is known that watercress was used in ancient Egypt and it has a long history of medicinal use. The ancient Greeks provided it to their soldiers for stamina and some African tribes believed it was an aphrodisiac.

Crisp and peppery, watercress has a real bite. It can be used in salads and soups and on sandwiches, and is often juiced to optimize its antibiotic properties. It is best to eat it fresh.

Other Foods for Breast Health

Other good anti-inflammatory foods are turmeric, onions and garlic. And just as for heart health, it is also important to eat plenty of omega-3s and not so much omega-6 oils to protect your breasts. Women whose diets are high in omega-3s have a lower breast cancer risk.

Another group of foods that inhibit or slow tumor growth contain a substance called apigenin. It is contained in many very common foods including parsley and celery, but can also be found in Chinese cabbage, bell peppers, apples, cherries, oranges, nuts and other plant products, as well as wine and tea.

Vitamin D and Breast Cancer

Vitamin D deficiency has been linked to everything from higher rates of caesarian section deliveries to obesity and osteoporosis. Rickets, once a major health concern in the U.S., has become rare since the

1930's, when milk began to be fortified with vitamin D.

Can vitamin D do for cancer, what it's done for rickets? A growing number of experts are convinced.

A study from Creighton University School of Medicine in Nebraska in 2007 concluded that supplementing with calcium and *vitamin D reduced the risk of cancer (including breast, colon and skin cancers) by 77%*.

Many other studies have linked vitamin D deficiency with diabetes, Alzheimer's disease, heart disease, auto-immune diseases, Parkinson's disease, depression and autism.

Vitamin D is a fat soluble vitamin which we (and most plants and animals) produce through exposure to the sun. Its major function in the body is to maintain normal blood levels of calcium and phosphorous.

The best way to get your vitamin D is through 10-15 minutes of exposure to the summer sun per day. This means actually peeling down and getting a good area of skin exposed **without sunscreen** since that blocks most vitamin D production.

Aside from sun exposure, the natural food sources for vitamin D include fatty fish (salmon, mackerel and sardines), liver and eggs. Milk, cereals and other processed grains are often fortified with vitamin D. However, most Americans don't (or won't) eat a sufficient quantity of those D-rich foods to get the minimum daily requirement.

What about in the winter? Anyone in the northern hemisphere will have to either find a good UVB tanning bed or take vitamin D supplements.

The government's recommended daily allowance for vitamin D has just been raised to about 600 units, which is only the amount necessary to avoid rickets but not enough to optimize health benefits. For that, Dr. Mark Hyman recommends a maintenance dosage of 2,000 to 4,000 units. However, if you think you need more, get tested by a doctor before increasing dosages.

Recent research concluded that daily intakes of vitamin D in the range of 4000-8000 IU are needed to maintain blood levels required to reduce by about half, the risk not only of breast cancer but also of colon cancer and multiple sclerosis.

Iodine and Breast Health

Another important nutrient in breast health is iodine. We talked a little about iodine in connection with thyroid and weight gain. It also has an estrogen connection. Here's how.

When iodine levels are low, the ovaries produce more estrogen and at the same time the estrogen receptors in the breast tissue increase their sensitivity. So more estrogen is produced and more is going to the breasts, which increases the risk for cancer.

It's important to take the iodine test described in Chapter 7 and if you are low consult with a holistic health care provider.

Xenoestrogens

As I said before, 80% of breast cancer is attributable to diet and environmental factors. Although it is primarily diet, we need to talk about the environmental factors and the most important of those are xenoestrogens.

Xenoestrogens are petrochemicals or substances made from petroleum oil. *Xeno* is the Greek word for stranger or foreigner so these substances are foreign to the human body.

Xenoestrogens have strong hormone-like or estrogen-like effects in our bodies. They are also known as endocrine disruptors because they wreak havoc with our hormonal system.

They behave like estrogen - in fact very potent estrogens, not like the weak phytoestrogens - because there is something in their molecular structure that allows them to fit into hormone receptors on each of our cells.

Xenoestrogens are even more potent than the estrogens that are produced by our ovaries.

Because they are made from petrochemicals, xenoestrogens are everywhere in our environment.

They are in millions of products from plastics, microchips, medicines, clothing, foods, soaps, pesticides and perfumes. They are in air pollution as well as water and soils.

They are in bug sprays, tub and tile cleaners, detergents, dishwashing liquids, cosmetics, toiletries, herbicides, fungicides and weed killers. They are in car exhaust, dry cleaning chemicals, and nearly all plastics.

Phthalates

Is your shampoo making you fat?

If you diet and exercise and your weight doesn't budge, you might want to check your medicine cabinet. Researchers from the Children's Environmental Health Center at The Mount Sinai Medical Center in New York found an association between a class of chemical substances known as "phthalates" and obesity in young children.

Phthalates are man-made chemicals that disrupt your endocrine system because they mimic the body's natural hormones. They are commonly used in building materials like plastic flooring and wall coverings, food processing materials and medical devices. They are also found in many personal-care products such as shampoos, nail polish, deodorants, fragrances, cosmetics, hair gels, mousses, hairsprays, and hand and body lotions. You'll also find them in varnishes and nutritional supplement coatings.

Phthalates have already been cited as a concern for menopausal women because of their endocrine disrupting properties. Previous studies have found that use of phthalates among pregnant women can lead to a feminization of boy babies and infertility in men. Animal studies suggest they can lead to breast cancer.

Organic Food: Should you or shouldn't you?

According to Dr. John Lee the entire planet is now "awash in a petrochemical sea of xenoestrogens." This, he says, has led to an epidemic of reproductive abnormalities, including cancers of the reproductive tract, infertility, low sperm counts and even the feminization of males.

Research shows that exposure to xenoestrogens suppresses the immune system. It also hampers T-lymphocyte function and natural killer (NK) cells. These are some of your strongest defenses against cancer.

Xenoestrogens are also fat soluble and non-biodegradable. That means that they don't break down in the environment, they just hang around. When they get into your fat cells, they just sit there.

This is another reason to be careful of the food you eat. Try to buy organic fruits and vegetables to minimize the amount of pesticides and other chemicals that come on your food.

The Environmental Working Group publishes the "**Dirty Dozen Plus**™," a list of the foods that are most important to buy in their organic versions because they are heavily treated with chemicals.

They also publish the "**Clean 15**™," a list of foods that are not heavily treated with chemicals, and so you may not need to buy organic versions. Here are the foods that made their most recent list of the worst and best:

ALWAYS BUY ORGANIC	*NO NEED TO BUY ORGANIC*
Peaches	Eggplant
Apples	Cabbage
Sweet bell peppers	Kiwi
Celery	Asparagus
Nectarines	Sweet peas
Strawberries	Mango
Cherries	Pineapple
Grapes (imported)	Sweet corn
Spinach	Avocado
Potatoes	Onion
Blueberries	Cantaloupe
Green beans	(domestic)
Collard greens	Watermelon
Kale	Grapefruit
	Honeydew melon
	Sweet potatoes

Also, be very careful of the animal products that you buy. If animals are eating pesticide-laden feed, those chemicals get stored in the animal's fat. You ingest those xenoestrogens when you eat the meat. They can then accumulate in your fatty tissues (brain, liver, and breast among others) and cause estrogen dominance that may lead to breast cancer.

This is another reason to buy only organic, grass-fed meat, free-range organic poultry and wild caught fish. All animal products should be hormone and anti-biotic free.

Solvents

Another category of xenoestrogens is solvents. These are used in industrial processes like automobile manufacturing and repair; paint and varnish manufacturing; electronics; industrial cleaning; and dry cleaning. Also, fingernail polish and remover, I'm sorry to say, falls into this category.

Symptoms of exposure to solvents include fatigue and depression, lack of coordination and inability to focus. Other effects are brain swelling (headaches), and oxygen deprivation in the brain with lowered cognitive abilities.

Over a longer period of exposure, solvents can cause mood disturbances such as depression, irritability, fatigue and anxiety as well as inability to focus, and short-term memory loss.

To minimize all these xenoestrogens it is advisable to:

1. Avoid the use of pesticides, herbicides or fungicides in gardening.

2. Check for toxic ingredients in cosmetics and toiletries and try to buy non-toxic versions. There are no non-toxic versions of hairspray or nail polish or polish remover available. Check the Environmental Working Groups list of safe personal care products.

3. Avoid fabric softeners.

4. Avoid most scented products, perfumes and air fresheners. Try natural aromatic oils or essential oils.

5. Try unscented laundry soaps and naturally scented shampoos and conditioners.

6. Use filtered water in place of tap or bottled water.

7. Avoid using plastic containers to the extent that you can, and don't drink from plastic cups.

8. Don't microwave in plastic containers or use plastic wrap when microwaving.

Recipe: Lemon Broccoli and Avocado

- 4 crowns of broccoli
- 1 avocado
- 1 lemon
- 1 tablespoon extra virgin olive oil
- 1/4 teaspoon unrefined sea salt and pepper to taste

Chop broccoli into bite-sized pieces and steam for 3 minutes.

In mixing bowl, combine juice from the lemon, the oil and the salt and pepper.

Chop the avocado into chunks and add to bowl. Add warm broccoli, mix gently and serve.

Recipe: Strawberry, Spinach and Sesame Salad

- 2 bags of pre-washed organic baby spinach
- 4 cups of fresh organic strawberries, sliced
- ½ teaspoon Dijon mustard
- ½ cup extra virgin olive oil
- ¼ cup white wine vinegar
- ¼ cup sesame seeds
- Coarse unrefined sea salt
- Coarsely ground black pepper

Whisk together the mustard, olive oil and vinegar. Add sesame seeds and salt and pepper to taste.

Pour dressing over spinach and strawberries and toss until well coated.

Chapter 8

Adrenal Support at Midlife

As we strive to balance our hormones in midlife it's important to understand how hormones are produced and how they might get out of whack.

You probably already know that progesterone is the hormone produced by the ovaries at the time of ovulation. Its name means "pro-gestation" and it supports pregnancy by supporting the egg through fertilization. Later it supports the development of the fetus.

Progesterone also has many other roles. It's a precursor to estrogen, meaning that the body uses progesterone to produce estrogen as well as testosterone and many of the stress hormones produced by the adrenal glands.

But the most common imbalance of hormones at menopause is an imbalance of estrogen and progesterone. Many symptoms result from an excess of estrogen relative to progesterone. How do these two get so out of balance? During menopause, progesterone drops an estimated rate that is 12 times the decline rate of estrogen.

When estrogen is too high relative to progesterone, the estrogen is said to be "unopposed." That means its effects are not counterbalanced by progesterone. Even if estrogen levels are lower at menopause, if it is unopposed by progesterone, even low estrogen levels may promote breast cancer and increase the risk of endometrial cancer. In addition, it can cause bloating and water retention, and disrupt electrolytes in the cells. All of this can contribute to mood swings, loss of concentration, and aches and pains.

So why don't women in underdeveloped countries report the same frequency of these problems during menopause? Dr. John Lee, in his book *What Your Doctor May Not Tell You About Menopause: The Breakthrough Book on Natural Hormone Balance*, proposes two possibilities. One is that women in underdeveloped countries are not as stressed out as Western women and so their adrenal glands are still functioning and able to produce progesterone at midlife. Secondly, they have a diet rich in phytochemicals or dietary sources of hormones that keep their hormone production levels higher.

Progesterone and Your Adrenal Glands

During your reproductive years estrogen and progesterone are produced by your ovaries. Long before you had your first period your body was producing those hormones but they were not being produced by the ovaries. Estrogen and progesterone were originally produced by your adrenal glands. You don't hear much about your adrenal glands but they are important for many different parts of your life.

The adrenals are two walnut sized glands that sit on top of your kidneys. When you go through puberty, the adrenals stop producing sex hormones (estrogen, progesterone and testosterone) and work full time managing your stress by, among other things, producing adrenaline and cortisol. Those are your stress hormones.

But when menopause comes around, your ovaries have had it and they stop producing sex hormones. That's a natural process that occurs as you run out of eggs. Then the job of producing those hormones goes back to the adrenal glands.

But if you are overly stressed, or if you have lived in a completely stress filled environment for years, your adrenal glands can be really tired – too tired to manage your stress, let alone go back to producing sex hormones.

The adrenal glands are capable of producing progesterone which as I said before is a precursor to estrogen and testosterone. But progesterone is also a precursor to the corticosteroids which manage our stress. If we are stressed, the body is going to use whatever progesterone it has to try to relieve that stress and there may be very little - or even none - left over to balance out estrogen levels.

How do you know if your adrenals are stressed, fatigued or even exhausted? Here are some of the most common symptoms:

- Excessive sweating from little activity
- Lower back pain
- Knee weakness or pain, especially on the side
- Dark circles under the eyes
- Dizziness
- Muscle twitches
- Low blood sugar
- Heart palpitations
- Sensitivity to light
- Difficulty seeing at night
- Salt cravings
- Low stamina for stress, easily irritated
- Excessive mood swings after eating carbohydrates
- Chronic infections
- Low blood pressure
- Feeling tired but wired
- Poor sleep
- Cravings for sweets and carbs, intolerance to alcohol
- Premature aging
- Dry skin with excessive pigmentation
- Lack of libido
- Cystic breasts
- Tendency to startle easily

If you want a healthy menopause, you need healthy adrenal glands and that means managing stress and nourishing your adrenals.

How do you nourish your adrenal glands?

To nourish your adrenals you need to eat whole, organic, natural, unprocessed foods. The adrenal glands get enormously overworked when they have to process sugar, sweets and refined starches. They simply can't keep up with the demand when a stressful diet is added to an already stressful life. For healthy adrenals, the first essential step is to avoid refined sugar and processed carbohydrates, caffeine and alcohol.

Another way to boost adrenal health is through cholesterol. As we've already seen, progesterone is a precursor to estrogen, but the precursor to progesterone is actually cholesterol. In fact, cholesterol is the most important raw material that your body needs to produce all of the hundreds of hormone in your body. It is the mother of all hormones. That's why there is no need to avoid butter, dairy, red meat and eggs.

But cholesterol has a gotten a bad reputation when it comes to heart health. We will be talking about the myth of cholesterol and your heart in Chapter 8.

Salt and the Adrenal Glands

You'll see from the list above that one of the common symptoms of adrenal fatigue is a craving for salt. This is because your body needs salt to support the adrenal glands. Many people have cut way back on salt thinking that it's necessary to lower blood pressure and be heart healthy. The truth, however, is that a low salt diet will just compound the problem of weak adrenal glands.

Even if they are not actually doing it, most Americans believe that reducing salt in their diets is a good, healthy and necessary thing. Doctors are all for it and the USDA 2010 Dietary Guidelines for Americans promote it. But there is an argument to be made that Americans really aren't eating too much salt and shouldn't be on reduced sodium diets.

Speaking recently at a press conference criticizing the USDA's Dietary Guidelines, Mort Satin, Vice President of Science and Research at the Salt Institute, which represents the salt industry, made the case for taste. He points out that while the Dietary Guidelines recommend increasing salad and dark green vegetable consumption, the general population needs some salt to get past the healthy, but bitter phytochemicals in them. He cites a broccoli study showing that reducing salt makes these foods less appealing, and without it green vegetables can "taste like grass."

Satin also points out that reducing salt intake may also exacerbate the obesity epidemic as people "consume more calories just to satisfy their innate salt appetite." He likens the situation to the introduction of 'light' beer, low-calorie soda and low-fat foods, all of which led people to eat or drink more of the engineered product. It is likely that consumers faced with low-salt potato chips will simple eat more because they are not getting what they are craving.

In general, according to Satin, Americans are eating less salt than ever. Until the 1950's when refrigeration became widespread, salt was the primary means of food preservation. Salt consumption dropped dramatically after that and today the levels of salt consumption in the Mediterranean diet, which is touted as healthy, have always been and currently are about 40% higher than in the US diet.

The Dietary Guidelines are recommending a level of salt far lower than can be found in any other country in the world and lower than in any period in recorded history, says Satin. He worries that the Guidelines "effectively place the entire population of the US into a massive clinical trial without the consumers' knowledge and certainly without their consent."

Satin points to "considerable peer-reviewed clinical research" predicting negative consequences for population-wide salt reduction." And while the Salt Institute has, for many years, repeatedly asked the Secretary of Health and Human Services to support a large clinical trial that would show the health outcomes resulting from population-wide salt reduction, the request has always been refused.

By ignoring available studies and refusing to conduct clinical trials, Satin concludes that the

Dietary Guidelines on salt are "confused, simplistic and far more a product of ideology than of science."

What kind of salt should you use?

The quality of the salt you use is key for good health. Do you buy regular refined table salt, sea salt, or unrefined sea salt? Here's what you need to know.

Salt can be mined in caves or it can be found in the sea. Most refined table salt is mined and then bleached and processed to be pure white and contain nothing but sodium and chloride.

But sea salt is produced by drying out salt from the sea. It too can be bleached white and processed. So it's not enough to say that you are eating sea salt.

Unrefined sea salt is the best choice. It should not be bleached white but retain its natural color which can range from yellow to pink to brown or even black. The color tells you that the salt has retained about 17 trace minerals from the sea that are good for us.

The best choices to look for are Celtic sea salt or Himalayan sea salt.

Salt and Iodine

While unrefined sea salt is great, the one thing that it is missing is iodine. Most table salt in the United States is iodized which means it has iodine added to it. This is considered one of the great public health triumphs of the 20th Century because since table salt began to be iodized in 1924, the problem of goiter was substantially eliminated.

Unfortunately, today the incidence of goiters is again on the rise. Goiter is a thyroid condition caused by insufficient iodine. The thyroid needs iodine to produce hormones. Signs of iodine deficiency may include a goiter, weight gain, cold intolerance, and fatigue. In pregnant women it can lead to miscarriage or mental retardation of the baby.

If you want to test yourself at home for iodine deficiency, here's how you do it. This is a simple test suggested by Dr. John Douillard, author of *The 3- Season Diet: Eat the Way Nature Intended*:

- Get a bottle of **2% iodine tincture** at the drugstore.
- With a Q-tip, paint a **2-inch square** on the **inside** of your forearm just below the elbow.
- **Let dry**. Don't bathe or swim until the patch fades.
- If the iodine patch fades away in **less than 10-12 hours** it indicates a need for increased iodine.

Learning to Eat Seaweed for Iodine

Most Americans only get iodine from their refined table salt. But you can and should get it from food.

Foods high in iodine include saltwater fish, shellfish, seaweed, kelp and kombu.

Kombu is a member of the kelp family and can be purchased dried, pickled or shredded. It is used in Japanese cuisine as a flavor enhancer and tenderizer. It's available in Asian food markets and also at health food stores.

According to Paul Pitchford, author of *Healing with Whole Foods: Asian Traditions and Modern Nutrition*, kombu is the only food that is an adequate source of the minerals that our bodies need. Those minerals are important as the foundation of all nutrients and no other nutrient will work in the body without minerals, since they are the basic structure for building proteins, enzymes and vitamins.

Dried kombu usually comes in dark green strips about one inch wide by seven inches long and expands greatly when soaked or cooked. It is a rich natural source of both sodium and potassium and a 3.5 inch strip provides more than 100% of the recommended daily value of iodine.

Cooking with kombu is simple. Just add a 3 or 4 inch strip to the pot when cooking any brown rice or other whole grain. The kombu will be cooked in 30 to 45 minutes and can then be sliced or diced into the grain or eaten separately.

Kombu can also be added to beans while they cook to tenderize them and make them more digestible. If cooked longer in a soup or a stew, the kombu will dissolve when stirred.

Eating kombu diced or sliced is something of an acquired taste. Pitchford recommends starting with a one inch strip and says that you have to eat if for several weeks before you develop the natural enzymes necessary to break it down and truly enjoy the flavor. The effort is worth it to ensure your supply of daily minerals.

Give kombu a try. While you develop a taste for it remember that other very good sources of iodine include yogurt, cow's milk, eggs, poultry, mozzarella cheese and strawberries.

Stress and Your Adrenals

We talked about boosting progesterone levels by supporting the adrenal glands through a whole foods diet.

The other way to reduce the burden on your adrenal glands is to decrease the stress in your life.

According to James L. Wilson, ND, PhD, author of *Adrenal Fatigue, The 21st Century Stress Syndrome*, adrenal fatigue occurs when stress from any source whether it's physical, emotional, mental or environmental, exceeds, either cumulatively or in intensity, the body's capacity to adjust appropriately to the demands placed upon it by the stress.

There are many ways to reduce the stress load on your adrenals and here are just a few:

- Positive thoughts, mantras or affirmations
- Guided imagery
- Meditation
- Keep a journal
- Laughter or smiling (even if you are faking it)
- Massage therapy
- More rest and better quality sleep – get to bed by 10 p.m.
- Personal down time every day
- Surround yourself with like-minded people
- Avoid people who drain your energy

Studies have shown that just putting a smile on your face has the same effect on your brain as 2,000 pounds of chocolate or receiving $25,000! So smile.

The Relaxation Response

A particularly easy and effective way to deal with stress is using the relaxation response. The relaxation response is the collective physiologic responses in your body that occur when you are in a state of meditation. But you don't actually have to be meditating to get the benefits. If you fool your body by acting *as though* you are in that state you can achieve the same benefits.

And the benefits of relaxation for your adrenals are great. During relaxation, the stimulation of your adrenal glands diminishes so they can rest. When this happens, all the tissues in your body become less sensitive to stress hormones so all parts of your body can recuperate.

Belly Breathing

One of the best ways to trigger the relaxation response very quickly is a simple deep breathing exercise.

Belly breathing is the way babies breathe and it is the most natural way for us to breathe. By expanding and contracting the belly, rather than the chest, the air can reach the lower part of the lungs where there is a rich blood supply.

The relaxation response can be triggered in just a few minutes of belly breathing.

Try it right now. Lie or sit comfortably with your full body supported. Place the palms of your hands on your abdomen, just below your navel. Close your eyes.

Imagine you have a balloon in your belly under your hands. As you inhale through your nose, imagine you are inflating the balloon and as you exhale, also through your nose, imagine you are deflating the balloon. Do not expand your chest.

If you want to add a positive mantra or affirmation to your belly breathing, that is good. Try "relax" or "peace" or "I am still" or "I open my heart" or "Om." Otherwise just concentrate on the air moving in and out.

Try doing this for five or ten minutes once a day.

Another good practice is just remembering to take a deep breath and release any tension you feel in your body periodically during the day but especially when you are having a hot flash. Let the hot flash be a reminder to do some deep breathing.

I am always surprised when I have a hot flash how much tension I am holding in my chest and when I release that tension and breathe, the flash passes much more quickly.

It is also great to do your breathing just before meals. According to psychologist and diet expert Marc David in his book *The Slow Down Diet: Eating for Pleasure, Energy & Weight Loss*, when we are stressed, our digestion turns off. Our bodies do not waste time digesting food when it thinks there is an emergency going on.

That's why if you rush your food because you're busy and want to get on to the next thing on your list, your food just sits like a rock in your stomach. Your digestion has been turned off.

But when we are in relaxation mode, our digestion is fully activated. And we can fool our bodies into thinking that we are in relaxation mode even if there is chaos all around us. By doing that belly breathing exercise before meals, your body will relax and turn on its digestion.

Try taking 10 belly breaths before eating just one meal a day and see if you notice the difference.

Recipe: Easy Fried Brown Rice

- 1 tablespoon olive oil
- 1 small onion
- 2 cloves garlic, minced
- 1 carrot, diced
- 1/2 bunch scallions
- 1 tablespoon grated ginger
- 4 cups cooked brown rice
- 1 egg
- 2 tablespoons tamari soy sauce

Saute onion and garlic, add carrots and cook for 4 minutes. Add scallions and ginger, saute for 4 more minutes. Add rice and sprinkle with water to generate steam.

Beat egg with tamari sauce and add mixture to pan, stirring it around quickly with a fork to scramble. Lower heat and cook for about 5 minutes, stirring occasionally.

Recipe: Gingered Greens Beans with Hijiki

- ½ cup dried hijiki seaweed
- 1 tablespoon organic tamari soy sauce
- 2 tablespoons extra virgin olive oil
- ½ cup onion, halved and sliced
- 2 tablespoons finely chopped garlic
- 3 tablespoons grated peeled fresh ginger root
- Pinch Celtic Sea Salt

Soak hijiki in hot water for about 30 minutes. Drain and rinse well in colander to remove any grit.

Combine hijiki in a saucepan with tamari sauce and water to almost cover it. Cook uncovered over medium heat until water has nearly evaporated, about 30-40 minutes.

While hijiki cooks, heat oil in skillet over medium-high heat. Add onion, garlic, and salt and sauté for about 4 minutes. Cut tips from beans, and add to onions. Cover and cook until beans are tender-crisp, about 3-5 minutes. Add hijiki and ginger. Mix well.

Serves 2-4.

From Alicia Silverstone's *The Kind Diet*

Chapter 9

Heart Disease and Menopause

The biggest health concern for menopausal women is heart disease. Cardiovascular disease is the number one killer of both men and women in the United States, and it affects one in four Americans.

The interesting thing is that the rate of death from heart disease has been declining in the past 20 years. That's the good news. The bad news is that it's only been declining for men. For women, heart attack deaths have been increasing.

Today 50% of women who have a heart attack will die of it. This is very concerning in itself, but what's even more alarming is that women are more likely to die of a first heart attack and have no previous symptoms.

One problem is that when it comes to heart disease, women are being treated like men and that just doesn't work.

Men have heart attacks because they accumulate plaque in their arteries and can have up to 90% blockage in their arteries. That blockage has probably grown over a long period of years starting in a boy's early teens.

Women don't have the same plaque buildup but may suffer a fatal heart attack with only 20-30% blockage in their arteries. Only 50% of women die with their major arteries blocked.

What is the real cause of heart attack in women? It's not a major blockage but a smaller blockage combined with spasms of the arteries or heart muscles. The spasms cause the *total* blockage of the artery.

Why are women suffering these spasms? According to Dr. John Lee in his book *What Your Doctor May Not Tell You About Menopause: The Breakthrough Book on Natural Hormone Balance* there are 4 main reasons:

- Bad fats and oils
- Low magnesium levels causing electrolyte imbalances
- High stress levels
- Conventional hormone replacement therapy

We talked before about good fats and bad fats and we will talk even more about them later.

We have also talked about stress in connection with digestion and hormonal balance but stress is also a critically important factor in connection with heart disease. Those same stress relieving strategies that we talked about in Chapter 7 will also support your heart's health. Remember to take time during the day to do some deep belly breathing.

Magnesium Deficiency and Heart Disease

Women who survive heart attacks have been found to have higher magnesium levels than those who die from the attack.

According to Paul Pitchford, author of *Healing with Whole Foods: Asian Traditions and Modern Nutrition*, magnesium is an essential mineral that activates over 350 processes in the body and supports harmonious flows within various systems. Without sufficient magnesium he says, we "get stuck" and this manifests as constipation and other digestive problems, irregularities in menstrual flow, problems with reproductive health, muscle spasms, and headaches.

Pitchford believes that about 70% of the U. S. population suffers from magnesium deficiency and that it is one of the most under-diagnosed mineral deficiencies. He is one of the original proponents of the benefits of whole foods and believes that by eating a diet of processed refined foods, we could be missing out on as many as 90 to 100 essential minerals, including magnesium.

To make matters worse, magnesium is depleted from our bodies by diuretic use, diabetes, alcohol, age and diarrhea.

The list of foods containing magnesium is a long one and it's relatively easy to remedy the deficiency. The foods that have the highest magnesium content are:

- dried seaweed
- chocolate (cacao)
- beans
- whole grains (especially buckwheat, millet, wheat berries, corn, barley, rye and rice)
- nuts (especially almonds, cashews and filberts)
- sesame seeds
- wheatgrass and barley grass
- spirulina and chlorella

Dairy, eggs, meat and fruit contain the least amount of magnesium.

Chocolate has a higher magnesium level than any other food except seaweed. Pitchford believes that most chocoholics have magnesium-poor diets and are craving the mineral to improve the health of their nerves and bones.

Eating dark chocolate with only wholesome ingredients (no hydrogenated fats or refined sugar) can contribute to a healthy mineralization of the body.

Heart Disease and Hormone Replacement Therapy

For more than 20 years, doctors looked at the rise in heart disease among women after menopause and concluded that it was caused by insufficient estrogen. That fueled the big push for hormone replacement therapy by the pharmaceutical industry. The problem is heart disease is not caused by insufficient estrogen.

It's true that estrogen has the effect of relaxing blood vessels and so it can protect against a heart attack. However, according to Dr. John Lee, 66% of women over the age of 65 have plenty of estradiol (one of several types of estrogen in our bodies) for this function.

The real issue is the proper balance of estrogen. Too little can cause problems but if you have too much estrogen, you could have a higher risk of developing blood clots and strokes.

Dr. Lee believes that increased heart disease after menopause is related to deficient levels of progesterone, not estrogen. The benefits of progesterone are:

- Increases the burning of fats for energy

- Reduces inflammation

- Protects the integrity and function of cell membranes

- Prevents loss of potassium and magnesium

On the other hand, the synthetic progestins contained in HRT (sold under the brand name Provera) increase the risk of arterial and heart spasms. So why are these synthetic hormones still on the market? Because they are huge moneymakers for the pharmaceutical industry. HRT is even bigger than tranquilizers, antibiotics and antidepressants.

Sugar and Heart Disease

Another big culprit in heart disease is sugar. The famous Framingham Study estimated that 60 percent of heart disease in women is caused by insulin resistance which is the precursor to Type 2 Diabetes.

The biggest problem with sugar is that it causes inflammation. And it is the inflammation in the body that leads to chronic diseases like heart disease, cancer and diabetes.

Keep in mind that when we talk about sugar, we're not just talking about the granulated white stuff. We're also talking about all kinds of sugar that are found in processed foods. Sugar includes things like Snapple, vitamin water, protein and energy bars, candies, cookies, crackers and most commercial yogurts.

Refined sugar contained in all of those products is an unreliable and insufficient source of energy. It wreaks havoc in our bodies disturbing normal insulin levels. It immediately enters your bloodstream giving you a rush of energy. But just as quickly its effects are gone and you feel deflated.

Our bodies have very little time to burn sugar and, unfortunately, what is not burned in that short amount of time turns to fat.

Even worse, in order to be processed sugar literally strips from our body

- calcium
- magnesium
- phosphate
- potassium
- sodium
- vitamin B6.

Basically it steals some of the most important nutrients our bodies need.

The American Heart Association only recently acknowledged the role of sugar in heart disease and issued guidelines for women to limit their added sugars to 6 or 7 teaspoons a day which is 24 to 28 grams. Keep in mind that 4 grams of sugar are equal to one teaspoon.

Yet on average, Americans consume 1 cup of refined sugar a day!

Natural Alternatives to White Sugar

What are some natural sweeteners we can use instead of refined table sugar?

Fruit is a great one. It has natural fiber that will slow down and reduce the absorption of sugar into the bloodstream.

Here is a list of other natural sweeteners all of which should be used in limited quantities.

Agave Nectar

Agave nectar is a natural liquid sweetener made from the juice of the agave cactus. It is 1.4 times sweeter than refined sugar.

Despite its reputation as a healthy sweetener, agave is high in fructose and some research suggests that fructose does not shut off appetite hormones, so you may end up overeating.

Xylitol

Also referred to as birch sugar, this natural sugar substitute can be made from tree fiber or corncobs, and occurs naturally in many fruits and mushrooms. Xylitol is sweet, yet low on the glycemic index, and can be used by those with diabetes and hypo-glycemia. It has 40% fewer calories than sugar. Studies show that it prevents tooth decay and repairs tooth enamel.

Brown Rice Syrup

This product consists of brown rice that has been ground and cooked, converting the starches to maltose. Brown rice syrup tastes like moderately sweet butterscotch and is quite delicious. In recipes, replace each cup of white sugar with ¼ cup brown rice syrup, and reduce the amount of other liquids. There is some glucose in brown rice syrup so diabetics should avoid using this sweetener.

There is some concern with the arsenic levels in brown rice syrup (and brown rice in general) since the publication of a study by Consumer Reports. The study found that most brown rice currently on the market is high in arsenic. For that reason, your use of brown rice syrup should be limited.

Honey

One of the oldest natural sweeteners, honey is sweeter than sugar. Depending on the plant source, honey can have a range of flavors, from dark and strongly flavored, to light and mildly flavored. Raw honey contains small amounts of enzymes, minerals and vitamins that have health and healing properties.

Maple Syrup

Maple syrup is made from boiled-down maple tree sap and contains many minerals. 40 gallons of sap are needed to make one gallon of maple syrup. It adds a pleasant flavor to foods and is great for baking.

Be sure to buy 100% pure maple syrup and not maple-flavored corn syrup. Grade B is stronger in flavor and said to have more minerals than Grade A.

Molasses

Organic molasses is probably the most nutritious sweetener derived from sugar cane or sugar beet, and is made by a process of clarifying and blending the extracted juices. The longer the juice is boiled, the less sweet, more nutritious and darker the product is. Molasses imparts a very distinct flavor to food. Blackstrap molasses, the most nutritious variety, is a good source of iron, calcium, magnesium and potassium.

Rapadura

This brand-name product is made from a process of extracting juice from the sugarcane plant, evaporating the water from the juice, and then grinding the results into a fine powdery texture. Rapadura is organic, rich in vitamins and minerals and unrefined.

Stevia

This leafy herb has been used for centuries by native South Americans. The extract from stevia is 100 to 300 times sweeter than white sugar. It can be used in cooking, baking and beverages, does not affect blood sugar levels, and has zero calories. Stevia is available in a powder or liquid form, but be sure to get the green or brown liquids or powders, because the white and clear versions are highly refined.

Sucanat

Short for Sugar Cane Natural, this brand-name product consists of evaporated organic cane juice made through a mechanical rather than a chemical process, and thus is less refined, retaining many of the sugarcane's original vitamins and minerals. It has a grainy texture and can be used in place of white sugar.

Erythritol

This sugar alcohol is a sweetener available in a powdered form. It is formed from the breaking down, fermenting, and filtering of sugar cane or corn starch. It has a cool taste that works well in coffee and tea. Erythritol doesn't affect your blood sugar or cause tooth decay. The drawback of this sweetener is that it may cause gas, bloating and diarrhea if consumed in excess.

Sugar alcohols (sorbitol, mannitol, xylitol, maltitol, erythritol and lactitol) are highly processed but considered natural. These are generally considered safe but may give rise to gastrointestinal problems.

This is not a list of sweeteners that you should be using on a daily basis. They are all to be used sparingly. Yes, they are better than refined sugar because they have retained vitamins and minerals. But we don't need that much concentrated sweet in our lives.

Concentrated sweeteners are for special occasions. Using them 4 or 5 times a day in coffee or tea adds up and can do damage in terms of weight gain, sweet cravings and unbalanced blood sugar levels.

Artificial Sweeteners

Many women want to use a sugar substitute or artificial sweeteners for weight control or blood sugar control. I only advocate natural sweeteners. But here is a list of artificial sweeteners and the drawbacks of each.

Sucrolose (Splenda). I don't recommend Splenda because there are just too many questions about it. If you use this or are thinking about it, I recommend that you read *"Sweet Deception: Why Splenda, NutraSweet and the FDA May be Hazardous to Your Health"* by Dr. Joseph Mercola. He points out that Splenda is not calorie-free but has 4 calories per envelope. In addition, it contains chlorine which is not only toxic but also a hormone disruptor. It's just not something you want to be putting into your body.

Aspartame (Equal, NutraSweet) and acesulfame. These have not been sufficiently tested. Aspartame breaks down to methyl alcohol (wood alcohol) in your body. For information about the possible risks of aspartame take a look at the documentary *"Sweet Misery: A Poisoned World."*

Saccharin (Sweet 'N Low). Despite the fact that saccharin has been removed from the list of cancer causing substances, it is still believed to increase risks of bladder cancer. Best to avoid it.

The Myth of Cholesterol and Heart Disease

If you watch TV at all you think cholesterol is the whole reason behind atherosclerosis and you also think that the cure is statin drugs like Zocor and Lipitor. The pharmaceutical companies are happy to have you believe this because the number one drug category in America is the statin drugs.

But what exactly is cholesterol and why is it under attack?

Cholesterol is a fatty substance produced by your liver that is needed for building and regulating your cells. It helps build your cell membranes, the covering layer of your nerves, and much of your brain.

Cholesterol is also a key building block for our hormone production, and without it you would not be able to maintain adequate levels of testosterone, estrogen, progesterone or cortisol.

Too little cholesterol is bad for you. In fact, you might be surprised to know that you can have too little cholesterol in your body. If cholesterol is too low, you could have problems with cell, nerve and brain function. You could also experience problems with hormone regulation. You might **also suffer with depression**.

You might be surprised to learn that people with the lowest cholesterol levels as they age are at the highest risk of death. According to Dr. John Lee, after the age of 65 there is no correlation at all between high cholesterol and heart disease.

In fact, if you use statins to try to force your cholesterol down after age 65, you do more harm than good. Higher cholesterol levels are actually associated with longer life spans.

What about before we get to 65? The problem is not the cholesterol but the fact that cholesterol can become oxidized or rancid, meaning that it can harden. But reducing the amount of cholesterol is not the answer. Removing the cause of the oxidation is.

Cholesterol can be ingested in the food we eat. Examples of foods that are high in cholesterol include foods that are high in fat such as red meat, and organ meats like liver and kidneys.

Other foods high in cholesterol include eggs, milk, cheese and other dairy products.

It's a myth that we have to reduce our dietary sources of cholesterol or eat a low-fat diet to reduce cholesterol and avoid heart disease. That's because most of your body's cholesterol is made in the liver and circulates in the bloodstream, where it does its work.

Watching the amount of cholesterol you consume – for example, by limiting the number of eggs you eat

- can have only a very small effect on your total cholesterol levels. You produce around 80-85% of your total cholesterol in your liver, using sugar, not fat.

That's right. It's mostly sugar again that is driving the levels of cholesterol and only 15-20% is made from cholesterol or fats that you are eating.

In the 1950's, at the time the American Heart Association was founded, there was a questionable study performed that associated cholesterol with heart disease. That study is the source of what is now known as the lipid hypothesis – the theory that fat causes heart disease.

The founder of the AHA was Dr. Dudley White who was also the personal physician to President Eisenhower. You may or may not be old enough to remember that President Eisenhower actually had 2 heart attacks while in office.

Dr. White strenuously disagreed with the hypothesis that dietary fat causes heart disease. He admitted that he did not understand the cause of the epidemic but was convinced it was not high fat foods like butter.

He reasoned that butter was around for hundreds of years and when he was in medical school in the early 1920's it was rare to see a heart attack.

In fact the first reported death from myocardial infarction was 1921 but by 1950 there were 400,000 cases. Today we have 700,000 cases of heart attack every year. But over the same time our use of butter has declined dramatically so it cannot possibly be the cause of heart disease.

Since 1926, consumption of butter has dropped precipitously, replaced by margarine and vegetable oils. At the same time cancer and heart disease have soared.

We do not have all the answers to what causes cancer and heart disease but for sure it's not the consumption of butter because these trends are going in the opposite direction.

Vegetable Oils

Since the early 20th century traditional saturated fats have been replaced by modern vegetable oils and these are compounding the problem of inflammation from our high sugar diets.

Let's just review the four types of fat:

- saturated fats,

- trans fats,

- polyunsaturated fats and

- monounsaturated fats.

Saturated fats usually come from animal products, such as meat, milk and cheese. It is referred to as saturated because of its chemical makeup and the fact that it has hydrogen atoms attached at all available receptors. It is therefore *saturated* with hydrogen.

For our purposes, the easiest way to know if a fat is saturated is whether in its natural state, it is solid at room temperature. A good example is bacon fat - it congeals when it's cooled, but you can melt it.

Saturated fat is found mainly in animal products, but is also found in some plant sources. Coconut oil and palm kernel oil contain saturated fat, for example.

Naturally occurring unsaturated fats, such as olive oil and corn oil, remain fluid at room temperature.

There are some benefits of saturated fats over unsaturated. For example, saturated fat is less likely to spoil or go rancid than unsaturated fat and is more stable during cooking.

Do we have to worry about saturated fat and heart disease?

Walter Willett, the head of Harvard Medical School's nutrition program has reviewed all of the research regarding fats and cardiovascular disease. He concludes that saturated fat raises the level of heart disease but in a very small way.

According to Dr. Willett saturated fat raises LDL levels — that's the so-called "bad" cholesterol - but it also raises the level of HDL or good cholesterol.

It is not so much the total level of you LDL but the level in relation to your HDL, that's important. If your LDL is high but your good HDL is also high, the ratio of the two may be good and not worrisome.

You have no doubt heard that eating red meat leads to heart attacks because of its saturated fat content. This is subject to serious debate and is unlikely to be true. Dr. John Lee discusses this in his book *What Your Doctor May Not Tell You About Menopause*.

His theory, backed by research from Harvard University, is that the inflammation related to red meat is actually caused by a vitamin B deficiency. Here's how that works.

When you eat red meat, which is a protein, it is broken down into amino acids, one of which is methionine. That in turn breaks down to homocysteine and finally to cysteine which is excreted by your body.

However, if the homocysteine is not broken down fast enough it causes an inflammation in the lining of the arteries leading to the plaque buildup that is a cause of arteriosclerosis and ultimately may lead to a heart attack.

According to Dr. Lee, if people with elevated homocysteine levels are given vitamins B6, B12 and folic acid, they reduce that risk. If you are deficient in those vitamins your body just accumulates the homocysteine rather than breaking it down and excreting it.

Food rich in vitamins B6, B12 and folate (vitamin B9) are on the following chart.

Food Sources of Heart Healthy B Vitamins	
Vitamin B6 (pyridioxine)	Bell peppers Turnip greens Spinach
Vitamin B12 (cobalamin)	Clams Calf's liver Trout Lamb Snapper
Folate (vitamin B9)	Spinach Parsley Broccoli Beets Turnip and mustard greens Asparagus Romaine lettuce Calf's liver Lentils

Trans Fats: The Most Dangerous Fat

Trans fat is a fake saturated fat that has disastrous effects on your heart and should be **eliminated entirely** from your diet.

Most of the trans fats that Americans consume are unsaturated or liquid oils that are transformed through a chemical process to a saturated or solid fat by adding hydrogen atoms. That chemical process is known as *hydrogenation* or *partial hydrogenation*.

Through the hydrogenation process, hydrogen is added to an oil like corn or soy oil to make it solid at room temperature, and convert it to something like margarine or shortening.

Partially hydrogenated oil was first produced about 100 years ago when chemists were looking for a cheap substance for making **candles**. They came up with something that resembled lard in appearance but was cheaper than lard or butter, and it caught on for baking.

The reason that products such as margarine and shortening were embraced by consumers and food producers was that they replaced fats which often became rancid and unstable. From a business standpoint, trans fat shortenings allowed convenience foods to be produced inexpensively, and with an increased shelf life. We wouldn't have aisles and aisles of packaged junk food today if it weren't for trans fats.

Early on everyone believed margarine was healthier than butter because of advertising, but researchers now know that the artificial trans fat in partially hydrogenated oil promotes heart disease through its effect on cholesterol.

Trans fat is much worse than any other kind of fat because not only does it raise bad LDL cholesterol, it also lowers good HDL cholesterol. It gives us a double whammy. It moves both types of cholesterol in the wrong direction.

The single most important thing to get out of your diet to avoid heart disease is trans fats. Researchers at the Harvard School of Public Health estimate that trans fat causes 72,000 to 228,000 heart attacks every year, including roughly 50,000 fatal ones.

All told, **artificial trans fat, on a gram-for gram basis, is the most harmful fat of all**. You should have **zero tolerance** for it in your diet and in your family's diet. **Adding just one gram of trans fat to your daily diet has been shown to increase the risk of cardiovascular disease by almost 85%**.

According to the U.S. Dietary Guidelines, Americans should eat less than 2 grams of trans fat per day. Even that is way too much. You should not be eating any at all. And yet **the average American adult has been consuming 5.6 grams of trans fats a day**.

How much trans fat are you consuming every day?

How do you even know if you're eating trans fats? You have to read the food labels. Trans fats must be disclosed on the label by law.

You will see a line for trans fats on all food labels. But beware. The government regulations permit food manufacturers to fudge the numbers.

If one serving of a product contains less than a half of a gram (.5 grams) of trans fat, the manufacturer is entitled to list zero trans fat and to advertise it as a trans fat free product. Those half gram servings of trans fats can add up quickly during the day and you may unwittingly exceed even the government's recommended level of 2 grams per day.

In addition, food companies can play games with serving sizes, making the serving size very small to get the trans fat number below .5 grams, even though consumers consider a serving size much more.

The only way to be sure there are zero trans fats in your diet is to **read the ingredient list**. If the words **"hydrogenated"** or **"partially hydrogenated"** appear on the ingredient list there are trans fats even if the package advertises "Zero Trans Fats."

Heart Disease and Polyunsaturated Fat

There are two kinds of unsaturated fats: mono-unsaturated and polyunsaturated.

Both polyunsaturated and monounsaturated fats help us by reducing risk of heart disease. They also build cell membranes, lubricate body surfaces, insulate us from the cold and carry the fat soluble vitamins A, D, E and K.

Fats are unsaturated when they have receptors that are missing hydrogen atoms. Monounsaturated fats are missing one hydrogen atom and polyunsaturated fats are missing multiple hydrogen atoms.

Monounsaturated fats are considered heart-healthy fats because they are typically a good source of the antioxidant vitamin E and reduce the risk of heart disease.

They can be found in:

- olives
- avocados
- hazelnuts, almonds, Brazil nuts, cashews
- sesame seeds, pumpkin seeds
- olive oil and peanut oil.

There are two types of polyunsaturated fats: omega-3 and omega-6 essential fatty acids. These fats are called essential because the body cannot produce them and we must get them through food.

Together, omega-3 and omega-6 fatty acids play a crucial role in brain function as well as normal growth and development. They are also necessary for stimulating skin and hair growth, maintaining bone health, regulating metabolism, and maintaining reproductive capability.

Susan Allport is a science writer and the author of *The Queen of Fats*. In her book she describes the essential difference between omega-3 and omega-6 fatty acids.

Omega-3s are found in plants but they are only found in the leaves of plants, so she refers to these fats as spring fats. They are what are produced in the spring when the whole world, both animal and vegetable, is coming alive and getting active. They are found in our bodies in those areas that are most active: eyes, hearts, brains and tails of sperm.

Omega-3s are the most abundant fats in the world but they are disappearing from our diets. They are the most abundant because they are found in phytoplankton (those microscopic green plants in the ocean) and in seaweed. We think of them as coming from fish but fish are rich in omega-3s only because they eat those greens.

Omega-3s regulate our brains, lower risk of heart disease, arthritis and cancer. They even help fight wrinkles and may block the formation of fat cells.

They are so essential to our lives that Harvard School of Public Health found that the absence of omega-3s in our diets is responsible for up to 96,000 premature deaths every year.

Omega-6 fats on the other hand are called the fall fats because they are found not in the leaves of plants but in the seeds. According to Allport, seeds are where plants store fat for the winter and when we eat seeds and the omega-6 fats, our bodies go into fat storage mode also.

These fats are slower and stiffer than omega-3s and promote blood clotting and inflammation, the underlying cause of many chronic diseases including heart disease and cancer.

Omega-3s and omega-6s are in competition to enter our cells and recently the blood-clotting, inflammation-producing omega-6s have been winning because there are so many more of them in our diet.

The foods that are high in Omega-3s (Alpha-Linoleic Acid) are:

- cold water fatty fish like salmon, mackerel and sardines
- herring, anchovy, lake or rainbow trout and tuna
- grass-fed beef and dairy products
- free range chickens and eggs
- seeds such as flax seed, chia seed, hemp seed, pumpkin seed
- walnuts
- dark leafy greens (kale, collards, parsley, wheat and barley grass)
- fish oil capsules

The foods that are high in Omega-6 (Linoleic Acid and Arachidonic Acid) include

- corn oil
- soybean oil
- cottonseed oil
- safflower oil and
- sunflower oil

Even if you don't think you use the omega-6 oils listed above, they are in processed foods in great quantity.

A healthy balance of omega-3s to omega-6s is 1:1. That means you should consume equal amounts of each or at the most, omega-6s could be about 4 times the amount of omega-3s. But the problem is that the average American consumes 40 times more omega-6s than omega-3s.

This imbalance between the two types of fats contributes to long-term diseases such as heart disease, cancer, asthma, arthritis and depression.

The increase in omega-6 use has occurred over the last hundred years as refining methods for pressing oil from seeds has been developed. Over a hundred years, we've increased our daily omega-6s from an average of 7 grams to 18 grams.

At the same time omega-3s have been disappearing from our food supply. Cows used to be grass-fed and produced meat, milk and cheese with higher levels of omega-3s. Chicken were free to roam and eat grass and bugs producing eggs and meat with higher levels. However, today cows and chickens are fed corn and soy making their meat and products full of omega-6s instead of the omega-3s.

A special note about salmon – only eat the wild caught, not farm raised salmon. When fish are raised in a farm, especially salmon, they are fed foods that are not natural for fish to eat. Salmon feeds on algae and on shell fish but on farms they are fed garbage, literally, as well as corn and soy. Those foods are not natural to the fish. These foods are high in omega-6 fats, which raises the omega-6 level of the fish and lowers the omega-3 level making them no longer the heart healthy fish that they are advertised as.

Canola oil is often advertised as rich in monounsaturated oil as well as omega-3 fats. However, canola oil is an engineered product from the rapeseed plant and there are many reasons to avoid it including the fact that it is rarely found in organic form, may be genetically modified and may contain trace amounts of hexane, an industrial toxin.

Eat more of the omega-3 rich foods, grass-fed, free-range and wild caught, and less of the other conventional meats. Use only olive oil and no vegetable oils whether it's corn, soy, sunflower or safflower.

Recipe: Steak with Brandy Cream Sauce

- 4 grass-fed tenderloin steaks
- 1 teaspoon unrefined sea salt
- 4 teaspoons coarsely ground black pepper
- 1 tablespoon butter
- 5 tablespoons cognac or brandy
- 3 tablespoons Dijon mustard
- 2/3 cup cream
- 2 tablespoons butter

Coat steaks with salt and pepper. Add butter to a hot pan, melt and add steaks. Turn once and cook to desired doneness. Remove and keep warm.

Add brandy to pan, let sit for 5 seconds and light with match. Flame should burn out after 10 seconds. Stir over medium high heat. Reduce heat to low and slowly stir in mustard and cream. Whisk in remaining 2 tablespoons of butter and stir until thick. Pour over steak.

From *The Liberation Diet*

Recipe: Black Bean and Avocado Salad

- 1/3 cup lime juice
- Zest of one lime
- ½ cup extra virgin olive oil
- 2 cloves garlic, minced
- 1 tsp. sea salt
- 1/8 tsp. cayenne pepper
- 2 (15 oz.) cans black beans, rinsed and drained
- 2 cups fresh corn kernels (or defrosted frozen kernels)
- ½ cup diced red onion
- 1 avocado, peeled, pitted and diced
- 1 yellow or orange bell pepper, diced
- 2 cups grape tomatoes, halved
- ½ cup chopped fresh Italian flat leaf parsley

Place lime juice, zest, olive oil, garlic, salt and cayenne in a small jar. Cover and shake until well combined.

Combine beans, corn, avocado, bell pepper, tomatoes, onion and parsley. Pour dressing over salad and stir gently until everything is well coated.

Chapter 10

Menopause and Bone Health

What is osteoporosis?

Why are we talking about bone health and osteoporosis in connection with menopause? Increasingly, bone health has become a concern for midlife women. If you want to live an active life into your 90's, standing straight and tall and even dancing, you want to protect your bones.

By 2020, it's estimated that 40 million women will be over 65 years of age and 20 to 30% of them will suffer a hip fracture before they are 90. Hip fractures are very serious because about 20% of people will die within a year as a result of the fracture and its complications. And half of those who don't die, never regain their mobility - they never walk again.

It is something of a myth that osteoporosis is a result of changes we go through in menopause. In fact, bone loss starts in our 30's and accelerates for a few years around peri-menopause and menopause, but then slows down again. Just because we are losing bone mass, however, doesn't mean that we should be having bone fractures. Those are two very different things.

Pharmaceutical companies emphasize the hardness of bones and the loss of bone density. They have defined bone loss as a disease. However, bone flexibility is the real key to avoiding fractures. We want bones that are both strong and flexible. We want bones that have some give and will bend but not snap.

Osteoporosis is also another one of those conditions that is not natural to the aging process but is a disease of modern lifestyles. In traditional cultures eating traditional foods, osteoporosis is unknown.

The Myth of Dairy and Strong Bones

When most people think about healthy bones, they think about calcium, and when they think about calcium they think about milk. But there is much more to bone health than dairy.

According to Annemarie Colbin, who wrote *The Whole-Food Guide to Strong Bones*, the fact is that in countries where people consume the most dairy, there are *higher*, not lower rates of bone fractures.

In addition, women who drink 2 glasses of milk per day have a *50% increased risk of breaking a hip* as those who drink one or fewer glasses.

It is not just dairy that's the problem. Calcium supplements are something that women are advised all the time to take and yet in a 1997 study, calcium supplements were associated with a ***doubling*** of the risk of hip fractures.

So what is going on? According to Dr. Colbin, it's true that calcium is a major mineral essential to bone health **but** it must be balanced. Too much calcium may make bones brittle, and brittle bones will shatter when hit.

About 65% of your bone mass consists of calcium phosphate which gives bones their hardness. The other 35% is a collagen matrix that gives bones their flexibility.

This collagen matrix that gives bones their flexibility is more important than calcium for preventing fractures because it helps bones bend rather than snap.

The medical community has focused on calcium intake and bone density to evaluate bone health but according to Dr. Colbin, there are 7 lifestyle risk factors that are much more accurate in predicting fractures:

1. Taking tranquilizers, including sleeping pills
2. Smoking
3. Vision problems such as poor depth perception
4. Being tall
5. Having a history of overactive thyroid
6. Having a high pulse rate
7. Being unable to rise from a chair without holding on to the arms

According to the 1997 study that I mentioned before, women having 5 or more of those risk factors had a 10% chance of breaking a hip in the next 5 years, while those with two or fewer had only a 1% chance.

Warning signs that you may have osteoporosis include:

- Sour taste in mouth in the morning (a sign of too much acid in your body)
- Dull, dry, brittle hair and thin, weak, peeling nails (a sign of too little protein)
- Gum recession and increased tooth loss
- Loss of height
- Chronic low back pain
- Leg cramps at night
- Restless behavior
- Insomnia
- Transparent skin
- Rheumatoid arthritis

The last 7 of these signs indicate a possible calcium or magnesium deficiency.

What are your wrinkles telling you about your bones?

A recent study finds that the worse a woman's skin wrinkles are during the first few years of menopause, the lower her bone density is. Researchers from the Yale School of Medicine believe that your skin may offer a glimpse of your skeleton's wellbeing.

The included 114 women in their late 40s and early 50s who had had their last menstrual period within the past three years and who were not taking hormone therapy. None of them had had cosmetic surgery.

The researchers scored the women for the number and depth of their wrinkles at the forehead and the cheek. They found that the worse a woman's wrinkles, the lower was her bone density. And conversely, women with firmer skin of the face and forehead had greater bone density. Why would that be?

According to the researchers, skin and bone share common building blocks in the form of proteins known as collagen. The same changes in collagen that lead to age related wrinkles and sagging skin, also contribute to the deterioration in our bone quality and density.

Ultimately, skin wrinkles may allow your doctor to assess whether you are more or less likely to fracture a bone without the expense of a DEXA scan.

How much calcium do you need?

A Swedish study recently confirmed that more calcium increases hip fractures. It found that women have the lowest risk of fracture when they consume about 750 mg of calcium per day. The U.S. government however advises women over 50 to take 1,200 mg per day. Just as a comparison, South African women have one-tenth the fractures of American women even though they take in half the calcium.

Not everyone needs the same amount of calcium especially when it comes to supplements. You have to look at your entire diet.

Dr. Colbin notes that if your diet is low in protein and sodium (both of which interfere with calcium absorption), it's quite possible that you only need 450 mg of calcium per day. Vitamin D and magnesium also affect how efficiently your body is using calcium.

And if you take calcium supplements in excess of what your body needs, you can have problems. Some women develop abdominal discomfort, constipation and even kidney stones. Many women are now developing something called the *calcium-alkali syndrome*. This is a dangerously high level of calcium in the blood and can lead to high blood pressure and kidney failure.

If you take more than 3,000 mg per day, you may have too much calcium in your blood, leading to another condition known as *hypercalcemia* which can lead to soft tissue calcification. This involves the accumulation of calcium in cells other than bone cells. In other words, you risk calcifying your tissues, joints, arteries, muscles and even your brain. It can lead to kidney stones and gall stones.

And there is worse news. A 2008 study found that taking calcium supplements for 5 years is associated with a 30% increase in heart attacks and higher rates of stroke and death in post-menopausal women. That study did not involve excess calcium, just any calcium supplements at all for 5 years.

The good news is that you are unlikely to overdose on calcium in your diet even though you might with supplements. If you are not careful with your diet, it can put you at risk for fractures. Here are some dietary habits to avoid:

- Eating too many refined, processed foods
- Eating a high proportion of **nightshade vegetables**
  - Potatoes
  - Tomatoes
  - Eggplant
  - Peppers
- Not eating enough leafy green vegetables
- Not eating enough protein
- Not having enough good quality fats in your diet

And maintaining a steady weight is also important. Women who lose 10% or more of their weight after age 50 have twice the risk of getting fractures.

Most Americans rely on dairy products to get their calcium. The USDA recommends 3 servings of dairy every day, thanks to the dairy lobby. But Dr.

Colbin points out that milk is one of 2 foods that make people sickest – the other one is sugar.

Dairy has been linked to coughs, colds, excess mucous, respiratory problems, ear infections, digestive disorders, female reproductive disorders, cysts, pimples, allergies and immune disorders.

And low fat dairy is even worse than full fat. You might think that 2% milk has 98% of the fat removed. That's not true. Whole milk is about 4% fat. So 2% milk is missing 50% of the naturally occurring fat.

Producers take out the fat but not any of the protein. That means low-fat dairy is too high in protein relative to fat. You need that fat to digest the proteins. Human milk is also about 4% fat and only 1% protein. Cow dairy is high in protein to build big hulking animals. Human milk is lower in protein, but relatively higher in fat to feed human brains rather than muscles.

If you are going to use dairy in your diet it's important to have only raw, unpasteurized products since during pasteurization the heat destroys not only bacteria, but also destroys vitamins, minerals and enzymes that are important for the digestion and assimilation of the milk.

Other Foods for Bone Health

But you really don't need dairy at all for healthy bones. Here is a list of non-dairy foods that are naturally high in calcium:

FOODS HIGH IN CALCIUM	
Cauliflower	Turnip greens
Watercress	Almonds
Parsley	Sesame seeds
Brussels sprouts	Pinto beans
Rutabagas	Sweet potatoes
Kale	Sardines
Mustard greens	Anchovies
Bok choy	Soft-shell crabs
Broccoli	Oysters

Olive Oil and Your Bones

Thanks to a pervasive advertising campaign involving white mustaches, most of us grew up convinced that milk is essential for building strong bones.

But according to a Spanish study involving olive oil, maybe we should be sporting greasy green-gold mustaches instead.

The two year study shows that eating a Mediterranean diet enriched with virgin olive oil is associated with increased serum osteocalcin con-centrations.

Osteocalcin is a protein secreted by osteoblasts, the body's bone building cells. Levels of osteocalcin in the blood are often used as a marker for bone formation. The higher levels found in this study suggest that olive oil may have a protective effect on bone.

Other studies have shown that osteoporosis rates within Europe are lower in the Mediterranean basin. Many researchers have speculated that the native diet could be the difference. The traditional Mediterranean diet is rich in fruits and vegetables, including olives and olive oil.

The Spanish researchers followed 127 men aged 55 to 80 years. Participants were randomly assigned to three different intervention groups. The first ate a typical Mediterranean diet with mixed nuts; the second group ate a Mediterranean diet with virgin olive oil, and the third group ate a low-fat diet.

Only the Mediterranean diet supplemented with virgin olive oil was found to be associated with a significant increase in total circulating osteocalcin and other bone formation markers.

In addition, participants following the other two diets were found to have lower serum calcium levels whereas those eating the olive oil had no significant changes in their calcium levels.

Olive oil: it does a body's bones good. Just not so good for dunking cookies.

Prunes and Bone Health

And there are other surprising foods that support bone health.

One Florida researcher found that prunes help prevent fractures and osteoporosis. He gathered 100 postmenopausal women and over a 12-month period, instructed one group of 55 women to eat 100 grams of dried plums (about 10 prunes) each day, while the second control group of 45 women ate 100 grams of dried apples.

The group that consumed prunes had significantly higher bone mineral density in the ulna (one of two long bones in the forearm) and spine, compared to the dried apple group.

According to the researcher, this was due in part to the ability of prunes to suppress the rate of bone resorption, or the breakdown of bone, which tends to exceed the rate of new bone growth as people age.

The researcher suggests eating two to three dried plums per day and increase gradually to perhaps 6 to 10 per day to get the full bone health benefits.

Other Nutrients for Bone Health

It's important to realize that calcium is not the only game in town when it comes to bones.

Calcium acts in a complex relationship with many other vitamins and minerals. For instance, calcium cannot be absorbed from the intestines to the bones without vitamin D, and it cannot be absorbed from the blood to the bones without magnesium.

Other nutrients that are important for building healthy bones are:

- Magnesium
- Vitamin D
- Vitamin C
- Boron
- Zinc
- Manganese
- Copper
- Vitamin K2

Why Osteoporosis Drugs Are Not the Answer

Many women are being prescribed drugs like Fosamax, Actonel and Boniva for osteoporosis but the side-effects are very disturbing. In fact those drugs may actually cause fractures.

The FDA warned consumers recently that there is a risk of a rare thigh bone fracture in people taking bisphosphonates. These are the drugs that slow or inhibit the loss of bone mass. The drugs have also long been associated with jaw necrosis, also known as *Fossy-jaw*, in which the jawbone crumbles. It is a horribly disfiguring condition.

Remember that your skeleton is a living organ. It is constantly replacing itself. In the two-stage process of bone remodeling, old bone must be broken down and lost, in order for new and stronger bone to be stimulated to grow and replace it.

Because bisphosphonates stop the breakdown or loss of (older) bone, they leave our bones somewhat denser but weaker. The new bone is built on older bone which is a weak foundation that can crumble. And that is exactly what happens.

The Power of Green Tea to Support Your Bones

Green tea is one of the latest superfoods making its way into bottled waters and energy drinks as well as energy bars, mints, chewing gum and even ice cream. It has many claimed benefits and some Texas research adds more evidence of osteoporosis prevention to the list.

Green tea is full of compounds called polyphenols which are known for their potent antioxidant activity.

Studies have shown that people who consume the highest levels of green tea polyphenols tend to have lower risks of several chronic degenerative diseases such as cardiovascular disease and osteoporosis.

Animal studies suggest that the mechanism behind this correlation may have to do with lowering chronic levels of inflammation.

Researchers at the Laura W. Bush Institute for Women's Health at Texas Tech University Health Sciences Center, focused on postmenopausal women and investigated the potential for green tea to work synergistically with tai chi in enhancing bone strength. Tai chi is a traditional Chinese form of moderately intense aerobic fitness activity grounded in mind-body philosophy.

In a double-blind, placebo-controlled, intervention trial 171 postmenopausal women with an average age of 57 years were divided into 4 groups:

- Placebo and no tai chi
- GTP: green tea polyphenols (500 mg/day) and no tai chi
- Placebo and tai chi (3 times/week)
- GTP+TC: green tea polyphenols and tai chi

The women in the study all had weak bones but not full-fledged osteoporosis.

The results showed that green tea polyphenols (at a level equivalent to about 4-6 cups of steeped green tea daily) improved bone health after 3 months and muscle strength at 6 months. In addition, participation in tai chi improved markers of bone health and muscle strength by 6 months.

The combination of green tea polyphenols and daily tai chi practice, however, also had substantial effects on markers of oxidative stress, which is the main precursor to inflammation.

The researchers believe that green tea and tai chi may help reduce the underlying cause of not only osteoporosis, but other inflammatory diseases as well.

Food Plan for Healthy Bones

To maintain strong and flexible bones naturally, a healthy diet is your best ally. Here are a few diet and lifestyle tips:

1. Eat dark green leafy vegetables every day to mineralize and alkalinize your body.

2. Eat sufficient protein to build the collagen matrix of bones. That's the 35% that gives you flexibility so bones bend and don't snap.

3. Make homemade soup stocks from bones. A great source of bone nutrients are the minerals found in the bones of other animals. We access those nutrients when we make soups that cook for hours. Slow cooking draws out the minerals from the bones and makes them available in a stock.

4. Spend 20-30 minutes a day in the sun and/or take a vitamin D3 supplement so that calcium is absorbed well and deposited to the bones and teeth.

5. Do some type of weight bearing exercise that also stretches tendons and muscles for bone building.

6. Quit smoking.

7. Cut down on alcohol and caffeine, which are also very acidic and can weaken bones.

8. Drink more green tea. Green tea combined with a daily tai chi practice was recently found to improve bone health in post-menopausal women.

Recipe: Chicken Bone Stock

- 1 whole free-range chicken
- 4 quarts cold filtered water
- 2 tablespoons apple cider vinegar
- 1 large onion, coarsely chopped
- 2 carrots, peeled and coarsely chopped
- 3 stalks celery, coarsely chopped
- 1 bunch parsley
- 6-7 inches of dried kombu

Cut chicken into several large pieces and place in a large stainless steel pot with water, vinegar, carrots, onion, celery and kombu. Let stand 30 minutes to an hour.

Bring to a boil and remove any scum that floats to the top. Reduce heat, cover and simmer for 6 to 24 hours. The longer the stock cooks, the richer it will be. About 10 minutes before finishing add the parsley, which adds additional minerals.

Remove chicken pieces with slotted spoon and reserve for other uses such as chicken salad or sandwiches.

Strain stock into a large bowl and refrigerate until fat rises to top. Skim off the fat and discard. Store stock in the refrigerator or freezer.

Adapted from *Nourishing Traditions* by Sally Fallon

Chapter 11

Menopause Superfoods

There are great foods for menopause and eating a whole foods diet of unprocessed, fruits, vegetables and whole grains, while indulging less in sugar, caffeine and alcohol, is a fantastic way to get a great foundation for a healthy menopause.

But if you want to take your health to a new level and feel not just like your old self, but *better than you have ever felt in your entire life,* then you want to tune into the power of superfoods for a **magnificent** menopause.

What are superfoods? In a nutshell, they are foods that have multiple health benefits.

David Wolfe wrote the most famous book on the subject called *"Superfoods: The Food and Medicine of the Future"* and he defines a superfood as something that has a dozen or more unique properties, not just one or two. Here's what he says:

> *Superfoods are both a food and a medicine; they have elements of both. They are a class of the most potent, super-concentrated, and nutrient-rich foods on the planet - they have more bang for the buck*

than our usual foods. ...
[S]uperfoods have the ability to
tremendously increase the vital
force and energy of one's body, and
are the optimum choice for
improving overall health, boosting
the immune system, elevating
serotonin production, enhancing
sexuality, and cleansing and
alkalizing the body.

Everyone has their own list of superfoods and I am going to share some of mine with you. Here are my top 7 superfoods for hormonal balance that will help you escape from the flames of hormone hell and let you breeze through menopause and beyond.

Maca

Maca is a root vegetable that has been cultivated in the Peruvian Andes for over 2,600 years. Growing at about 10,000 feet above sea level, it is the highest altitude crop in the world.

Today, maca is enjoying a resurgence in popularity after almost becoming extinct in the 20th century. The new interest in maca grew from the research of Gloria Chacon de Popovici, Ph.D., a Peruvian biologist, who conducted studies beginning in the 1960's showing that maca increases fertility in rats, dogs, guinea pigs, rams, cows and yes, humans.

Ancient cultures and especially the Incans considered maca a superfood that improves energy, stamina and libido. Today, it usually grabs headlines for its aphrodisiac qualities and its reputation as a natural Viagra.

Maca Beats Stress

Maca is a menopause superfood because it is a powerful adaptogen. An adaptogen is a nutritive substance that counters adverse sources of stress and allows the body to adapt naturally to stressful conditions. Adaptogens also help improve the body's natural balance or homeostasis.

According to David Wolfe, maca

> *"increases energy, endurance, oxygen in the blood, physical strength, neurotransmitter production, and libido. It supports the endocrine system, the adrenals, and the thyroid, typically improves one's mood, and helps support healthy hormone production."*

You can see how maca can be a superfood for menopausal women.

Maca has been recommended for everything from impotence and infertility to depression, hot flashes, stress and memory loss.

How does maca work?

It works its magic by stimulating the hypothalamus and pituitary glands which in turn regulate the other glands in the body and can bring balance to the adrenal, thyroid, pancreas and ovarian glands.

Typically dried and powdered, maca is rich in calcium, magnesium, phosphorous, potassium, sulfur, sodium and iron as well as vitamins B1 (thiamin), B2 (riboflavin), C and E. It also contains zinc, iodine, copper, manganese and silicon. Compared to the potato which also originated in the Andes, maca contains five times more protein and four times more fiber.

Maca has a butterscotch scent but a slightly funky turnip flavor that can be a little strong for some people. Don't let that stop you. You can take 1 or 2 tablespoons per day, and even more if you like, because studies have shown no toxicity or pharmacological effects.

You can add it to smoothies, salad dressings, soups, broth, tea or coffee.

Make sure you get the organic, raw and dried, powdered root. A good brand is Navitas and you can find it at health food stores, Whole Foods or at Amazon.com.

Chia Seeds

You remember those chia pets that were the rage when today's menopausal women were just kids? They are those clay figures with seeds that sprout a green coating of vegetation. Those seeds are also a superfood.

In ancient Aztec culture, chia seeds were a dietary staple as well as a valuable currency. They were carried by Aztec warriors for energy and endurance and it's said that one teaspoon fueled them for the entire day.

Chia seeds have a natural gel forming property which allows them to absorb up to 12 times their volume in water. If you mix a spoonful of chia seeds in a glass of water and let it stand for 30 minutes, the glass will contain a very thick gelatin. This is due to the high amount of soluble fiber in chia, which has one gram per tablespoon in addition to 4 grams of insoluble fiber.

The soluble fiber in chia seeds slows down the digestion of carbohydrates and their breakdown into sugar, keeping the blood sugar stable and helping to control or prevent diabetes. It also helps to rid the body of excess estrogens.

Weight Loss and Chia

By absorbing water and expanding, chia seeds contribute to a feeling of fullness which keeps appetite down and aids in controlling weight. The seeds also create bulk and improve elimination, keeping you regular.

And because they absorb liquid, chia seeds help to keep you hydrated and balance your electrolytes.

If you happen to be one of those people who just can't stomach fish, even though you know it's so healthy, here is some more good news. Chia seeds are the richest source of omega-3 fats, containing almost twice as much as fish.

Chia Seeds and Bone Health

But it doesn't stop there. Chia seeds also support bone health. One tablespoon contains 60 mg of calcium which is great, but even better, it provides the trace mineral boron, another catalyst for the absorption and utilization of calcium by the body.

You can add a tablespoon of chia seeds to your smoothie but drink it right away before the gel-producing qualities make it too thick to drink. Also sprinkle it on yogurt, cereal, oatmeal or salads.

Chia seeds are gluten-free and you can also add them to pancakes, muffins, breads or other baked goods.

When buying chia seeds make sure you get the organic versions. Navitas is a reliable brand and you can find them in health food stores, Whole Foods Markets and also on-line at Amazon.com.

Coconut Water

If you crack open a coconut, the clear juice that runs out is coconut water (not to be confused with coconut milk) and it's the latest rage in sports drinks. It's a superfood because it miraculously has the same electrolyte balance as human blood.

A proper balance of electrolytes is necessary for regulating blood pressure and for muscle co-ordination, heart and nerve function and concen-tration, all important for midlife women.

This makes it a better choice for rehydrating after a strenuous workout in hot weather or during an illness involving vomiting or diarrhea.

It is so naturally aligned with our bodies' com-position that during World War II in the Pacific coconut water was used as intravenous hydration and for emergency plasma transfusions.

Because it rebalances electrolytes it is also helpful for hangover relief the morning after. (So good to know!)

Coconut water contains all of the essential electrolytes including magnesium, sodium, phos-phorous and calcium, and is higher in potassium than most sports drinks, and even higher than bananas.

It has about 15 grams of natural sugar per serving but no processed sugars, unlike most sports drinks that have as much as 14 grams of processed sugar including high fructose corn syrup.

Coconut water doesn't really taste like coconuts but more like almonds. It has a mineral taste. Drink it plain or you can mix it with orange juice or your daily pomegranate juice, or use it in smoothies instead of water. Vendors are also producing flavored versions including tangerine, pineapple, acai and passion fruit, which might be a good way to begin experimenting.

Definitely chill it before drinking to improve the taste and it's very refreshing.

You can find it at Whole Foods Markets and health food stores as well as some major grocery chains. You can also order it on-line from Amazon.com. Some good brands are Vita Coco and O.N.E.

Sea Salt

Most health-conscious people are cutting down on their salt intake but that's not really the best choice for everyone.

Unless you have been diagnosed with high blood pressure and directed by a doctor to reduce your salt, there is good reason to add a high quality salt to your diet.

We have natural taste receptors on our tongue for salty foods and there is a good reason for that. If we don't get enough salt, we die.

Low-salt diets can even lead to weight gain. When we don't get enough salt we may have cravings for it because it provides essential minerals to our bodies. If we don't eat salt or if we eat primarily low sodium foods, we may continue to eat more and more calories trying to satisfy our innate salt appetite. Just as people eat too many low-fat cookies, we might eat too many low-sodium chips.

Before the 1950's when refrigeration became widely available, salt was the primary means of preserving food. But the government has been advising us to cut way back on the amount of salt that we eat to about 1,500 mg per day. Even the healthy Mediterranean diet is 40% higher than that.

Food would taste terrible without some salt. Salt actually helps us eat healthy foods. Try eating broccoli without salt. It would discourage even the biggest health nut.

Risks of Low-Salt Diets

Cutting down on salt can be hazardous to your health. Lower sodium levels are actually associated with an increased risk of cardiovascular death. Low-salt diets lead to higher rates of cardiac events and to death.

Low-salt diets are also linked to an increase in insulin resistance, a precursor to Type 2 Diabetes.

Also, elderly patients with low sodium levels have more falls and broken hips and decreased cognitive abilities.

Quality Counts

Quality makes a big difference when you are choosing salt. Refined table salt has been stripped of all minerals and bleached white. That mineral deficiency in your salt can create a mineral deficiency in your body that may manifest as a craving for salty pretzels, chips and nuts. If you add unrefined, unbleached sea salt to your diet, those cravings will diminish.

Also remember that salt cravings can indicate that our adrenal glands, so important for hormonal balance, are out of whack and need salt.

Finally, unrefined sea salt can actually help us detoxify our bodies from certain poisons that are everywhere in our environment. Dr. David Brownstein points out that our environment is full of toxins called halides which include fluoride and bromide (found in bread!). Both of these can raise the risk of breast cancer in the absence of healthy iodine levels.

To detox your body, Dr. Brownstein recommends iodine supplementation, plenty of water, vitamin C and unrefined sea salt. He advises 1 – 1 ½ teaspoons per day as a detoxing agent.

The best salt is unrefined Celtic Sea Salt which you can find at many health food stores.

Himalayan Pink Sea Salt is another good choice which you can buy on Amazon.com.

Broccoli Sprouts

Vegetables like broccoli contain a special chemical I mentioned before called sulforaphane which improves the liver's ability to detoxify carcinogens and other toxins.

Broccoli is high in sulforaphane. But broccoli **sprouts** are even more powerful than any other cruciferous vegetables. They contain *10 to 100 times higher levels of sulphoraphane* than regular broccoli. One *ounce* has as much of the active ingredient as one and a half *pounds* of broccoli!

What makes broccoli sprouts so powerful?

The sprouts have an abundant supply of the enzyme myrosinase that activates the sulphoraphane.

Researchers at Johns Hopkins University have developed a line of broccoli sprouts under the brand name BroccoSprouts. They are available in Whole Foods Markets, Wegman's Markets and other supermarkets.

They are great on a peanut butter sandwich or in vegetable spring rolls, or on top of a salad.

Pomegranates

Modern women at midlife have many options when it comes to dealing with nasty menopausal symptoms like mood swings, depression, bone loss, and fluctuating estrogen levels. But their most surprising and multi-tasking source of natural relief may come from an ancient food: the juicy pomegranate.

Pomegranates have been cultivated for over 4,000 years. Our word pomegranate dates back to around 750 B.C. and comes from the Latin *"Punicum malum"* meaning "Phoenician apple." Today the fruit is often called a "Chinese apple."

Despite its frequent comparison to an apple, the pomegranate bears a striking resemblance to the female ovary. It's not too surprising, then, that it served as a symbol of fertility for the Zoroastrians and other ancient cultures.

Fruits in general are defined as "the developed ovary of a seed plant" but in the case of the pomegranate fruit, the physical resemblance to a human female ovary is striking. Looking at a cross section of each reveals how similar are the containers for the pomegranate's seeds and the ovary's eggs.

But the pomegranate's resemblance to the female ovary goes beyond its physical similarities. The fruit also provides the same estrogens as the female ovary – estradiol, estrone and estriol.

What does this mean for a menopausal woman? It may very well mean relief from depressive moods and a lower risk of osteoporosis, breast cancer and heart disease.

Bone Loss Reversed

In an interesting 2004 study in the Journal of Ethnopharmacology, rats who had their ovaries removed suffered accelerated bone loss, a typical symptom of menopause.

When they were fed an extract of pomegranate juice and seeds for just 2 weeks, however, their bone mineral loss reverted to normal rates.

Mood Improvement

The same Japanese researchers in the 2004 study also found that the rats given pomegranate extract measured lower levels of depression indicators. Based on their results the authors found it conceivable that pomegranate would be clinically effective for women exhibiting a depressive state.

Heart Health

The rate of death from coronary heart disease in women after menopause is 2 to 3 times that of women the same age before menopause. **Here again, pomegranates provide proven healing benefits:**

Lowers Cholesterol - A 2000 study found that pomegranate juice is rich in antioxidants which prevent LDL (bad) cholesterol from oxidizing and leading to atherosclerosis.

Lower blood pressure - A small 2004 clinical study by Israeli researchers concluded that drinking one glass a day of pomegranate juice lowered blood pressure.

Blood clotting – One study in the Journal of Medicinal Foods showed that pomegranate juice slows down platelet aggregation and thins blood, preventing clotting.

Improves coronary heart disease – Several different studies have found that cardiovascular health is improved with the use of pomegranate juice since it reduces plaque, increases nitric oxide, and may prevent plaque from building in the arteries in some patients.

Increases oxygen flow - A 2007 study showed that drinking eight ounces of pomegranate juice daily for three months increased oxygen flow to the heart muscle in coronary patients.

Breast Cancer

Lab studies have shown pomegranate antho-cyanidins (sugarless plant pigments), flavonoids, and oils exert anticancer effects against breast tumors.

Although some women worry that foods with estrogenic properties may increase the risk of breast cancer, that isn't the case for pomegranates. In fact, pomegranate is a natural adaptogen, increasing levels of estrogen when the body is low but blocking stronger estrogens when levels are too high. This innate intelligence to adapt its function to the body's needs is an incredible benefit that natural foods have over pharmaceuticals.

In fact, pomegranate extract was compared to the drugs Tamoxifen and Estradiol in a 2011 study in the Journal of Nutritional Biochemistry. The researchers suggested that pomegranate extract may potentially prevent estrogen-dependent breast cancers.

How do pomegranates work their magic?

An 8 ounce glass of pomegranate juice contains about 40% of the RDA of vitamin C, and also is rich in vitamins A and E and folic acid.

The pomegranate fruit contains antioxidants called phytochemicals, which protect plants from harmful elements in the environment. These same phytochemicals when ingested protect the cells in our body. The juice has been found to contain higher levels of antioxidants than most other fruit juices, including cranberry or blueberry, and more even than red wine or green tea.

Drink the juice or eat the seeds (yes, they are edible) to reap the benefits of this menopause miracle. The seeds are available dried and sweetened and you can just throw a handful on top of salads or into your yogurt. You can find them at specialty stores, some supermarkets or online at Amazon.com.

Chocolate (Raw Cacao)

No list of superfoods would be complete without chocolate and it gets a lot of good press for its health benefits.

Dark chocolate has been proven to relieve emotional stress, lower blood pressure, improve blood flow by reducing platelet aggregation, lower cholesterol and improve cardiovascular health. It has been proven to lower the risk of stroke and heart attacks, both of which are big concerns for midlife women.

Part of that heart healthy effect comes from the high levels of magnesium in chocolate.

Magnesium also pushes calcium into our bones so it is important for bone health and preventing osteo-porosis.

Chocolate contains a substance called epicatechin which is also found in tea, and it has been proven to protect the brain in the event of a stroke. It also has substances called polyphenols which increase your good HDL cholesterol.

Sometimes we forget, but **chocolate is a vegetable**. It contains flavonoids which are antioxidants that resist or repair damage caused by free radicals formed by (a) normal bodily processes or (b) exertion or (c) environmental contaminants.

Raw and Unprocessed

The more chocolate is processed the more the flavonoids are destroyed. So the best source of chocolate antioxidants comes from dark chocolate (70% or higher) and an even better source is 100% raw cacao.

Raw cacao is available as beans, nibs, or powder and has the *highest concentration of antioxidants of any food*.

Smoothies are a great way to get cacao into your diet without adding in the sugars and milk solids that detract from its healthful benefits.

A good brand of the cacao powder is Navitas which is available in health food stores, Whole Foods Market and Amazon.com.

Is Red Wine a Superfood?

Red wine really doesn't qualify as a superfood but it does have some very healthful properties you should know about.

Red wine famously contains resveratrol, a compound found in the skins and seeds of red grapes. It's also found in peanuts, by the way. Resveratrol has been shown to protect the brain against the effects of a stroke.

Red wine is also a good source of a compound called catechins which could help raise levels of the good HDL cholesterol.

But it's not just red wine that gives you the benefits. Even champagne has the same polyphenol antioxidants that have been found to reduce the damage caused by free radicals. These antioxidants also reduce the release of nitric acid from the blood which keeps blood pressure down and reduces the risk of stroke and heart disease.

But it's important not to exaggerate the benefits of wine when we talk about menopausal women.

According to Walter Willett, head of Harvard's School of Public Health, much attention has been given to red wine but really what the science shows is that a daily drink of any kind of alcohol (including beer, white or red wine, or whiskey or other liquor) when you are over the age of 50 will reduce cardiovascular risk.

BUT the alcohol only has that effect if you have sufficient levels of folic acid in your body. That comes from taking folic acid supplements or eating foods rich in folate. Folic acid is a synthetic form of folate which is a B vitamin found in fruits and vegetables.

In order to get the heart benefits, women can have one drink a day but not two.

But if you do drink for the heart benefits you also have to be concerned about breast cancer risk because having just one drink *every other day* increases women's risk of breast cancer by 17%.

This puts women in a bind because they can help their heart but at the expense of their breasts. Here again, however, folic acid is important and the risk is minimized for women with high folic acid levels.

So if you drink, make sure that you are getting some good folate in your diet. The best sources are leafy greens, fruits, dried beans and peas.

Recipe: Raw Cacao Smoothie

- 1 cup coconut water
- 1 frozen banana
- 2 tablespoons raw cacao powder
- 1 tablespoon raw maca powder
- 1 tablespoon coconut oil
- 1 teaspoon cinnamon
- 1 tablespoon raw honey
- 2 tablespoons ground flax seeds or chia seeds

Add all ingredients to blender or Vitamix and blend until smooth. Enjoy!

Recipe: Raw Chocolate Mousse Parfait

Vanilla Cream

- ¼ cup water
- 1 cup raw cashews, soaked for 2-4 hours and drained
- ½ cup raw agave nectar
- 2 tablespoons organic vanilla extract

Combine all ingredients in a high speed blender. Blend to a fine sheen. Set aside to thicken.

Chocolate Mousse

- 2 tablespoons water
- 1 avocado
- 1 cup raw cacao powder
- ½ cup raw agave nectar
- ½ cup turbinado sugar
- 1 tablespoon organic vanilla extract
- ½ teaspoon cinnamon

- 3 cups diced strawberries

Combine all ingredients except cacoa powder in a high speed blender. Pour into a bowl and fold in cacoa powder.

In individual parfait or dessert glasses, layer vanilla cream, ½ cup diced strawberries and chocolate mousse. Chill before serving.

Resources

Books

Johnna Albi and Catherine Walthers, <u>Greens, Glorious Greens: More Than 140 Ways to Prepare All Those Great-Tasting, Super-Healthy, Beautiful Leafy Greens</u>

Edward Bauman, MEd, PhD and Helayne Waldman MS, EdD, <u>The Whole-Food Guide for Breast Cancer Survivors: A Nutritional Approach to Preventing Recurrence</u>

Kevin Brown, <u>The Liberation Diet: Setting America Free From the Bondage of Misinformation!</u>

Annemarie Colbin, Ph.D., <u>Food and Healing</u>

Annemarie Colbin, Ph.D., <u>The Natural Gourmet</u>

Annemarie Colbin, Ph.D., <u>The Whole-Food Guide to Strong Bones: A Holistic Approach</u>

Louann Brizendine, M.D., <u>The Female Brain</u>

Dr. David Brownstein, <u>Iodine: Why You Need It. Why You Can't Live Without It.</u>

Dr. David Brownstein, <u>Salt Your Way to Health</u>

Kaayla T. Daniel, PhD, The Whole Soy Story: The Dark Side of America's Favorite Health Food

Marc David, The Slow Down Diet: Eating for Pleasure, Energy and Weight Loss

Kathleen DesMaisons, Potatoes, Not Prozac: Solutions for Sugar Sensitivity

Dr. John Douillard, The Three Season Diet: Eat The Way Nature Intended

Mary G. Enig, Know Your Fats: The Complete Primer for Understanding the Nutrition of Fats, Oils and Cholesterol

Mary G. Enig and Sally Fallon, Eat Fat, Lose Fat: The Healthy Alternative to Trans Fats

Louise L. Hay, Power Thought Cards

Louise L. Hay, Self-Esteem Affirmations (CD)

Louise L. Hay, You Can Heal Your Life

John R. Lee, M.D., What Your Doctor May Not Tell You About Menopause: The Breakthrough Book on Natural Hormone Balance

Dr. Joseph Mercola, Sweet Deception: Why Splenda, NutraSweet and the FDA May Be Hazardous to Your Health

Sally Fallon, Nourishing Traditions: The Cookbook That Challenges Politically Correct Nutrition and the Diet Dictocrats

Leigh Anne Jasheway-Bryant, Not Guilty by Reason of Menopause

Christiane Northrup, M.D., The Wisdom of Menopause: Creating Physical and Emotional Health and Healing During the Change

Pamela Peeke, M.D., MPH, Fight Fat After Forty

Paul Pitchford, Healing with Whole Foods: Asian Traditions and Modern Nutrition

Joshua Rosenthal, Integrative Nutrition

Julia Ross, M.A., The Mood Cure: The 4-Step Program to Take Charge of Your Emotions--Today

Mary J. Shomon, The Thyroid Diet: Manage Your Metabolism for Lasting Weight Loss

Gary Taubes, Good Calories, Bad Calories: Fats, Carbs and the Controversial Science of Diet and Health

Gary Taubes, Why We Get Fat and What To Do About It

Kristina Turner, The Self-Healing Cookbook: Whole Foods to Balance Body, Mind and Moods

James L. Wilson, ND, DC, PhD, Adrenal Fatigue: The 21st Century Stress Syndrome

Susan Allport, The Queen of Fats: Why Omega-3s Were Removed from the Western Diet and What We Can Do to Replace Them

David Wolfe, Superfoods: The Food and Medicine of the Future .

Films

Food, Inc.

Food Matters

Menopause and Beyond: New Wisdom for Women

Rocky

Sweet Misery: A Poisoned World

The Gods Must Be Crazy

The Oiling of America

What the Bleep Do We Know!?

Websites

Sweet Nothings from the Center for Science in the Public Interest (http://www.cspinet.org/nah/05_04/sweet_nothings.pdf)

Printed in Great Britain
by Amazon

33559795R00126